P9-DHI-176

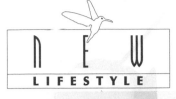

NEW
LIFESTYLE

Foods
that
Heal

George D. Pamplona-Roger, M.D.

*Author of the 'Encyclopedia of Medicinal Plants' and the 'Encyclopedia of Foods and Their Healing Power'
published in English, French, German, Portuguese, Italian, and Spanish*

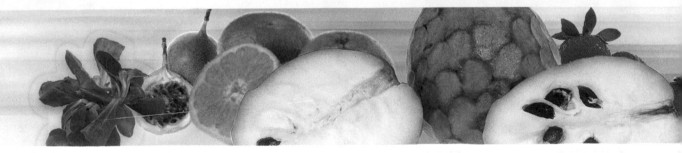

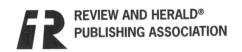

**REVIEW AND HERALD®
PUBLISHING ASSOCIATION**

editorial safeliz

Copyright © 2004 by **REVIEW AND HERALD PUBLISHING ASSOCIATION**
55 W. Oak Ridge Drive
Hagerstown, Maryland 21740
Phone: (301) 393 3000
e-mail: info@rpha.org – www.reviewandherald.org

ISBN 0-8280-1864-2

PRINTED IN THE UNITED STATES OF AMERICA

Editorial and Design by the editorial team of Safeliz S.L.
All drawings, images and pictures are owned by Editorial Safeliz S.L.

This magabook is an excerpt of the ENCYCLOPEDIA OF FOODS AND THEIR HEALING POWER,
published in three volumes by Editorial Safeliz S.L., ISBN 84-7208-184-2.
Copyright © 1995 by Editorial Safeliz S.L.
Pradillo, 6 – Polígono Industrial La Mina
28770 Colmenar Viejo, Madrid, Spain
Phone [+34] 918 459 877 – Fax [+34] 918 459 865
e-mail: admin@safeliz.com – www.safeliz.com

All rights reserved. **No part** *of this book may be transmitted or reproduced in any form or by any means, electronic or mechanical, including photocopying and recording, or by any information storage and retrieval system,* **without permission in writing** *from the publisher.*

Disclaimer: It is the wish of the author and the publisher that the contents of this work be of value in orienting and informing our readers concerning the nutritional, preventive, curative and culinary value of foods and recipes. Although the recommendations and information given are appropriate in most cases, they are of a general nature and cannot take into account the specific circumstances of individual situations. The information given in this book is not intended to take the place of professional medical care either in diagnosing or treating medical conditions. Do not attempt self-diagnosis or self-treatment without consulting a qualified medical professional. Some foods and products may cause allergic reactions in sensitive persons. Neither the publisher nor the author can assume responsibility for problems arising from the inappropriate use of foods by readers.

Foods
that
Heal

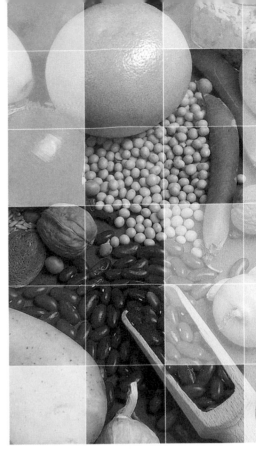

Table of Contents

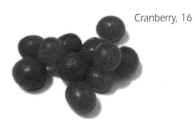

Cranberry, 16

Pasta, 25

Pomegranate, 80

5

Explanation of the pages describing specific foods

Icons indicating level of acidity or alkalinity of a food

Acidifying food: This is a food that, when metabolized in the body, produces acidification (**lowers the pH**) of the blood and other body fluids. **Cured cheese, meat, fish,** and **eggs** are the most acidifying foods.

Alkalizing food: This is a food that, when metabolized in the body, produces alkalization (**increases the pH**) of the blood and other body fluids. Fruit, together with vegetables are the most alkalizing foods. Because of this they protect against the acidification that is naturally produced within the body and aggravated by the consumption of foods of animal origin.

Icon for the botanical portion of the plant used as food.

Chapter title

Icon for the primary medical indication for the food or nutrient.

Icons for other medical indications.

Scientific name is the scientific denomination of the plant species that produces the food.

Common name Is the most widely used for the food described.

Subtitle Highlights the primary characteristics of the food.

Primary text

Graph of food composition (see p. 9, item 7)

Graph of fatty acids This displays the percentage distribution of the fatty acids that make up the fat content of the food. This graph is omitted for foods whose fat content is negligible, such as fruits and vegetables

Graph displaying composition of a food indicating the proportional distribution of the primary components as a % of total weight).

Photograph of the food described

Preparation and use This box includes both dietetic and culinary advice leading to improved utilization of the healing properties of the food.

Reference number Each method of preparation and use is assigned a reference number, which is used in the primary text to refer to the information in the Preparation and Use box.

Synonyms and description Scientific and common synonyms and botanical description of the species that produces the food.

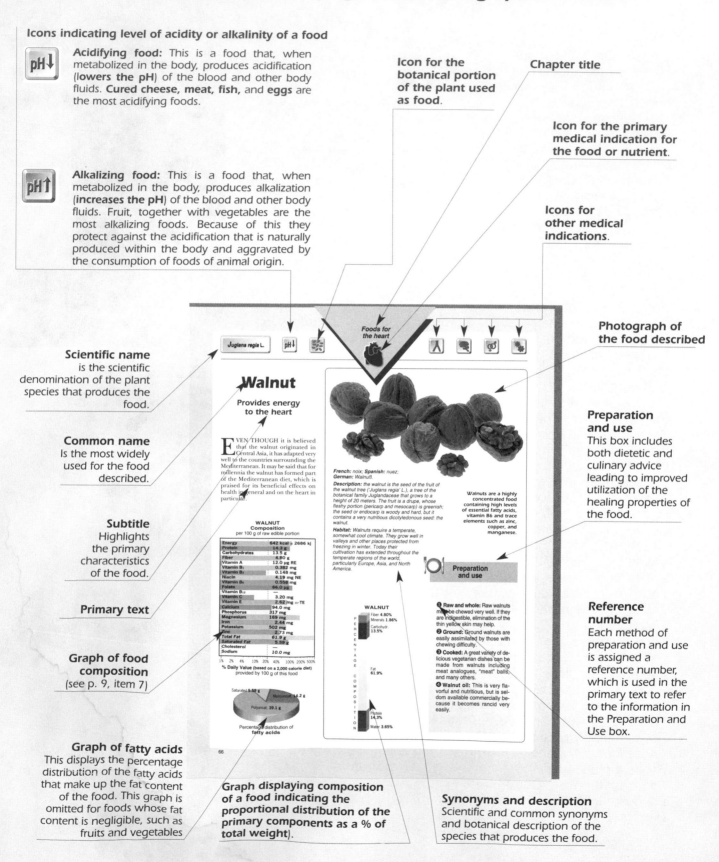

Walnut
Provides energy to the heart

Juglans regia L.

Foods for the heart

EVEN THOUGH it is believed that the walnut originated in Central Asia, it has adapted very well to the countries surrounding the Mediterranean. It may be said that for millennia the walnut has formed part of the Mediterranean diet, which is praised for its beneficial effects on health in general and on the heart in particular.

French: *noix;* **Spanish:** *nuez;* **German:** *Walnuß.*

Description: the walnut is the seed of the fruit of the walnut tree ('Juglans regia' L.), a tree of the botanical family Juglandaceae that grows to a height of 20 meters. The fruit is a drupe, whose fleshy portion (pericarp and mesocarp) is greenish; the seed or endocarp is woody and hard, but it contains a very nutritious dicotyledonous seed: the walnut.

Habitat: Walnuts require a temperate, somewhat cool climate. They grow well in valleys and other places protected from freezing in winter. Today their cultivation has extended throughout the temperate regions of the world, particularly Europe, Asia, and North America.

Walnuts are a highly concentrated food containing high levels of essential fatty acids, vitamin B6 and trace elements such as zinc, copper, and manganese.

WALNUT
Composition
per 100 g of raw edible portion

Energy	642 kcal = 2686 kJ
Protein	14.3 g
Carbohydrates	13.5 g
Fiber	4.80 g
Vitamin A	12.0 µg RE
Vitamin B₁	0.382 mg
Vitamin B₂	0.148 mg
Niacin	4.19 mg NE
Vitamin B₆	0.558 mg
Folate	66.0 µg
Vitamin B₁₂	—
Vitamin C	3.20 mg
Vitamin E	2.62 mg α-TE
Calcium	94.0 mg
Phosphorus	317 mg
Magnesium	169 mg
Iron	2.44 mg
Potassium	502 mg
Zinc	2.73 mg
Total Fat	61.9 g
Saturated Fat	5.59 g
Cholesterol	—
Sodium	10.0 mg

1% 2% 4%   10% 20% 40%   100% 200% 500%

% Daily Value (based on a 2,000 calorie diet) provided by 100 g of this food

Saturated 5.59 g
Monounsat. 14.2 g
Polyunsat. 39.1 g
Percentage distribution of **fatty acids**

WALNUT
Fiber 4.80%
Minerals 1.86%
Carbohydr. 13.5%
Fat 61.9%
Protein 14.3%
Water 3.65%
PERCENTAGE COMPOSITION

Preparation and use

❶ **Raw and whole:** Raw walnuts must be chewed very well. If they are indigestible, elimination of the thin yellow skin may help.

❷ **Ground:** Ground walnuts are easily assimilated by those with chewing difficulty.

❸ **Cooked:** A great variety of delicious vegetarian dishes can be made from walnuts including meat analogues, "meat" balls, and many others.

❹ **Walnut oil:** This is very flavorful and nutritious, but is seldom available commercially because it becomes rancid very easily.

66

Meaning of icons used in this work for medical indications

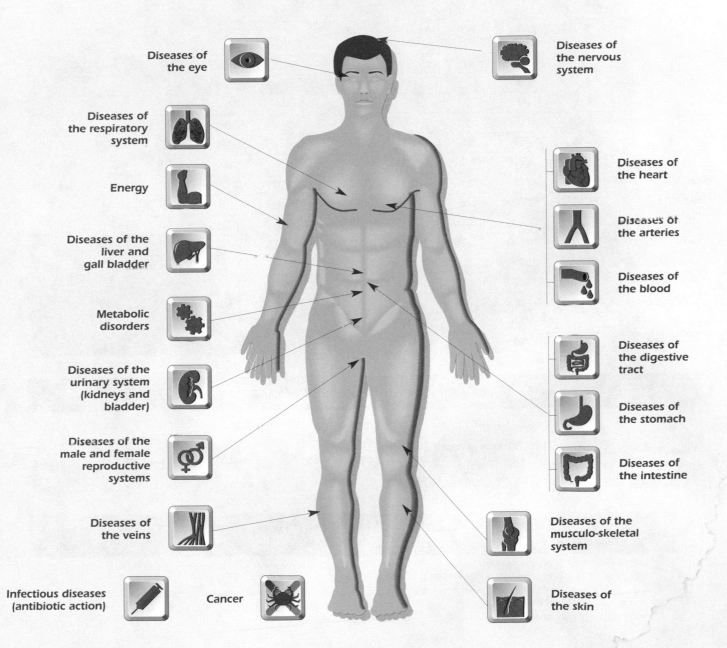

Diseases of the eye

Diseases of the nervous system

Diseases of the respiratory system

Energy

Diseases of the liver and gall bladder

Metabolic disorders

Diseases of the urinary system (kidneys and bladder)

Diseases of the male and female reproductive systems

Diseases of the veins

Infectious diseases (antibiotic action)

Cancer

Diseases of the heart

Diseases of the arteries

Diseases of the blood

Diseases of the digestive tract

Diseases of the stomach

Diseases of the intestine

Diseases of the musculo-skeletal system

Diseases of the skin

Recommended Daily Allowances (RDAs)
According to the National Academy of Sciences

Age		Proteins[1]	Vitamin A	Vitamin D[8]	Vitamin E	Vitamin K[8]	Vitamin C	Vitamin B₁	Vitamin B₂	Niacin	Vitamina B₆
		g m/f[2]	µg RE[3] m/f	µg[4] m/f	mg α–TE[5] m/f	µg m/f	mg m/f	mg m/f	mg m/f	mg NE[6] m/f	mg m/f
0 - 6	months	9.1	400	5	4	2.0	40	0.2	0.3	2	0.1
7 - 12	months	13.5	500	5	5	2.55	50	0.3	0.4	4	0.3
1 - 3	years	13	300	5	6	30	15	0.5	0.5	6	0.5
4 - 8	years	19	400	5	7	55	25	0.6	0.6	8	0.6
9 - 13	years	34/34	600/600	5/5	11/11	60/60	45/45	0.9/0.9	0.9/0.9	12/12	1.0/1.0
14 - 18	years	52/46	900/700	5/5	15/15	75/75	75/65	1.2/1.0	1.3/1.0	16/14	1.3/1.2
19 - 30	years	56/46	900/700	5/5	15/15	120/90	90/75	1.2/1.1	1.3/1.1	16/14	1.3/1.3
31 - 50	years	56/46	900/700	5/5	15/15	120/90	90/75	1.2/1.1	1.3/1.1	16/14	1.3/1.3
50 - 70	years	56/46	900/700	10/10	15/15	120/90	90/75	1.2/1.1	1.3/1.1	16/14	1.7/1.5
>70	years	56/46	900/700	15/15	15/15	120/90	90/75	1.2/1.1	1.3/1.1	16/14	1.7/1.5
Pregnancy ≤18 y.		71	750	5	15	75	80	1.4	1.4	18	1.9
Pregnancy >18 y.		71	770	5	15	90	85	1.4	1.4	18	1.9
Lactation ≤18 y.		71	1,200	5	19	75	115	1.4	1.6	17	2.0
Lactation >18 y.		71	1,300	5	19	90	120	1.4	1.6	17	2.0
Base for graphs[7]		**63**	**1,000**		**10**		**60**	**1.5**	**1.7**	**19**	**2.0**

Daily Fiber and Potassium Needs

	Children	Adults
Fiber	Amount calculated by multiplying the child's age by one gram for children between the ages of 5 and 10	Between 20 and 35 grams (average 25g; about 0.9 ounces)
Potassium	From 500 to 2,000 mg	2,000 mg

Acceptable Daily Intake (ADI)
of certain food components

Certain food components are harmful to health when ingested in excess. For this reason an ADI (Acceptable Daily Intake) has been established for each, which should not be exceeded in a healthful diet.

In contrast to many of the nutrients having a recommended daily allowance, the problem with these food components is their excess in the diet and not their lack.

In the graphs of the composition of each food, these components are shown in italics.

	ADI
Total fat	An amount that represents less than 30% of total caloric intake (approximately 65 g or 2.3 oz for a 2,000 calorie diet).
Saturated fat	An amount that represents less than 10% of total caloric intake (approximately 20 g or 0.7 oz for a 2,000 calorie diet).
Cholesterol	Maximum: 300 mg
Sodium	Maximum: 2,400 mg, which is equivalent to 6 grams (1/5 oz) of common table salt.

# of Nutrients
of the United States *

Age		Folates[9]	Vitamin B₁₂	Calcium	Phosphorus	Magnesium	Iron	Zinc	Iodine[8]	Selenium[8]
		µg m/f	µg m/f	mg m/f	mg m/f	mg m/f	mg m/f	mg m/f	µg m/f	µg m/f
0 - 6	months	65	0.4	210	100	30	0.27	2	110	15
7 - 12	months	80	0.5	270	275	75	11	3	130	20
1 - 3	years	150	0.9	500	460	80	7	3	90	20
4 - 8	years	200	1.2	800	500	130	10	5	90	30
9 - 13	years	300/300	1.8/1.8	1,300/1,300	1,250/1,250	240/240	8/8	8/8	120/120	40/40
14 - 18	years	400/400	2.4/2.4	1,300/1,300	1,250/1,250	410/360	11/15	11/9	150/150	55/55
19 - 30	years	400/400	2.4/2.4	1,000/1.000	700/700	400/310	8/18	11/8	150/150	55/55
31 - 50	years	400/400	2.4/2.4	1.000/1,000	700/700	420/320	8/18	11/8	150/150	55/55
50 - 70	years	400/400	2.4/2.4	1,200/1,200	700/700	420/320	8/8	11/8	150/150	55/55
>70	years	400/400	2.4/2.4	1,200/1,200	700/700	420/320	8/8	11/8	150/150	55/55
Pregnancy ≤18 y.		600	2.6	1,300	1,250	400	27	12	220	60
Pregnancy >18 y.		600	2.6	1,000	700	350	27	11	220	60
Lactation ≤18 y.		500	2.8	1,300	1,250	365	10	13	290	70
Lactation >18 y.		500	2.8	1,000	700	310	9	12	290	70
Base for graphs[7]		200	2.0	800	800	350	10	15		

* NATIONAL ACADEMY OF SCIENCES. *Dietary Reference Intakes for Calcium, Phosphorous, Magnesium, Vitamin D, and Fluoride (1997); Dietary Reference Intakes for Thiamin, Riboflavin, Niacin, Vitamin B6, Folate, Vitamin B12, Pantothenic Acid, Biotin, and Choline (1998); Dietary Reference Intakes for Vitamin C, Vitamin E, Selenium, and Carotenoids (2000); and Dietary Reference Intakes for Vitamin A, Vitamin K, Arsenic, Boron, Chromium, Copper, Iodine, Iron, Manganese, Molybdenum, Nickel, Silicon, Vanadium, and Zinc (2001).*

1. These amounts of proteins are calculated using the average weight of inhabitants of the United States for each age group. However, protein demand can also be calculated based on total caloric intake. In this case proteins necessary for an adult must provide the 10% of total caloric intake. The amounts derived in this manner are generally lower than those indicated in the National Academy of Sciences table.
   For example, a male between the ages of 31 and 50 years of age should ingest 56 g of proteins according to the table. But if his lifestyle is sedentary and he eats a 2,000-calorie daily diet, 50 g of protein is sufficient (10% of 2,000 kcal is 200 kcal in the form of proteins, which is obtained from 50 g. Each gram of protein provides 4 kcal).
2. m/f = male/female.
3. 1 µg RE (1 microgram of retinol equivalent) = 3.33 IU of vitamin A.
4. 1 µg of vitamin D = 40 IU.

5. 1 mg α-TE (1 milligram of alpha- tocopherol equivalent) = 1.5 IU of vitamin E.
6. The mg NE (milligrams of niacin equivalent) measure the preformed niacin found in foods in addition to that formed in the body from the amino acid tryptophan, which is found in the proteins in foods (60 mg of tryptophan transforms to 1 mg of niacin).
7. The amounts of this row are the RDAs given by the National Academy of Sciences for males between 25 and 50 years, as published in 1989. In this work, these amounts have been taken as the base for the calculation of the composition of foods' graphs. The percentages of the RDA of each nutrient provided by 100 g of foods, represented by colored vertical bars in the composition of foods' graphs have been calculated with the amounts of this row (see p. 6).
8. Vitamins D and K, iodine, and selenium are shown in this table. However, the are not included in graphs and tables showing the composition of foods for two reasons:
   • There is no reliable data concerning their content in many of the foods described in this magabook.
   • Their content in foods varies a great deal according to the composition of the soil where the foods were grown.

FOODS FOR HUMANS

With the exception of mother's milk during infancy, no food by itself provides all of the nutrients needed by humans. Therefore, knowing how to select foods and appropriately combine them is of vital importance.

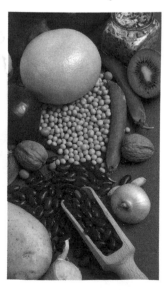

HUMAN BEINGS can eat just about anything as food, from mammary secretions (milk) to mineral crystals (common salt), including fruits, flowers, seeds, stalks, leaves, roots, seaweed, fungus, eggs of fish and birds or the dead bodies of various animals.

All of these, processed to a greater or lesser degree, provide thousands of different foods to the market.

Does the fact that we can eat this whole variety of foods mean that *all of them are equally fit for human consumption? Is there an ideal diet for humans that, in addition to being nourishing, maintains health and prevents disease?*

Chance or Intelligent Plan

The engineer has finished his work. The shining engine he has built is sitting on the test bench ready to be started for the first time.

"Here is the type of fuel that must be used in this engine", says the engineer to his assistants, "No other will give optimal results. And don't forget the oil. It must be exactly of this type!"

Only the one who has planned and built a engine can knowledgeably prescribe the type of fuel and lubricant the mechanism needs.

Specifically Recommended Foods

And is it not this way with humans? If human presence on planet Earth is just a random and unexpected consequence of evolutionary chance, then there should not be any particularly ideal foods. Man would have simply adapted to whatever foods were available, and whatever those might have been, they would have provided good health and wellbeing.

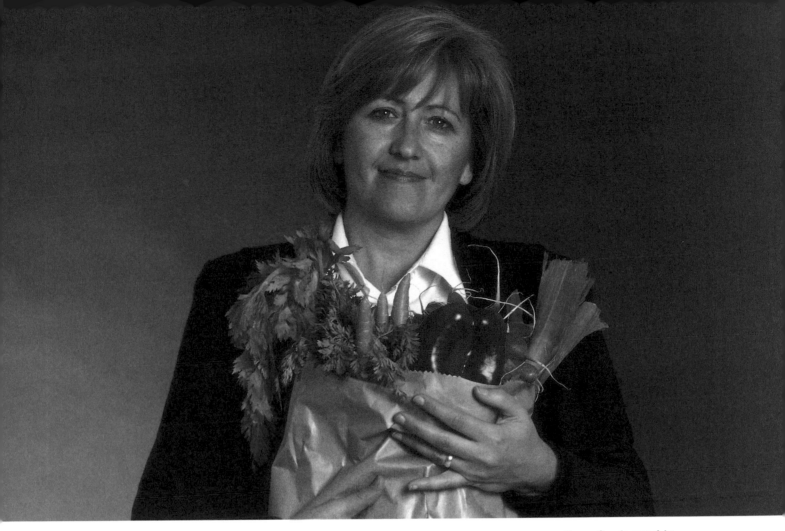

However, if humans were created by a superior Intelligence according to a specific plan and for a particular purpose, there should be, as well, specially created foods to maintain optimal physiological performance. Many believers find answers to these questions in the first chapters of Genesis, where it says that plants that bear seeds, **grains,** and, in a broader sense, **legumes, fruit** from trees[1] and **vegetables** that were added later,[2] constitute the *ideal diet* for the human species.

Adaptation, Yes, but Not by Eliminating Necessary Foods

Humans possess great capacity to adapt physiologically to many different types of foods. In spite of this, nutrition science has demonstrated that there are certain foods that *cannot be eliminated,* such as **fruit** and **fresh vegetables.** Not just any diet can produce good health. No matter how well we adapt to certain foods that are not ideal, such as those of animal ori-

gin, we continue to need vegetables, which are the most healthful and suitable. For example, Alaskan Eskimos have adapted to a diet rich in fish but they suffer a number of chronic diseases due to low consumption of fruit and vegetables.[3]

Some foods provide curative and preventive substances in addition to nutrients. Because of these benefits, foods that are well chosen and carefully used can cure, relieve and prevent many disorders and diseases.

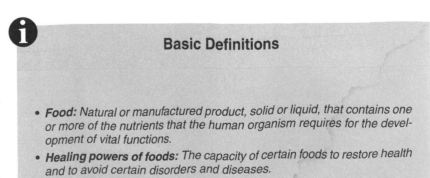

Basic Definitions

- **Food:** Natural or manufactured product, solid or liquid, that contains one or more of the nutrients that the human organism requires for the development of vital functions.
- **Healing powers of foods:** The capacity of certain foods to restore health and to avoid certain disorders and diseases.

11

What to expect from foods	Is this met by foods of vegetable origin?	Is this met by foods of animal origin?
That they will do no harm such as infections, poisoning, or other diseases. *Primum non nocere* (First, do no harm) is the old medical aphorism.	**Yes,** in general.	***Not*** always. They contain pathogenic **viruses, bacteria, and parasites at a** *much higher* **rate than vegetables.** ***Habitual* consumption** of some foods is *related* to **cancer** and **cardiovascular disease.**
That they provide the **energy** needed by the organism to function.	**Yes,** basically through carbohydrates (recommended).	**Yes,** primarily through proteins and fats.
That they supply needed **nutrients.**	**Yes,** *except* in the case of **vitamin B12;** although for reasons that are not well understood, strict vegetarians do not suffer from this lack as might be expected.	***Not completely.*** They provide *little* or ***no* vitamin C, vitamin E, carbohydrates** or cellulose ***fiber.***
That they **prevent or cure** disorders and diseases.	**Yes.** They have healing and preventive properties.	**No,** except in **very specific cases.**
That they provide a sense of **pleasure** when eaten	**Yes.**	**Yes.**

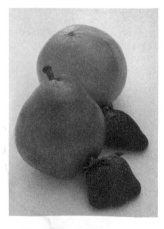

Fruits, grains, legumes as well as vegetables are particularly rich in antioxidants and accompanying substances known as phytochemical elements, that act as true natural pharmaceuticals.

Vegetable Foods, Source of Health and Healing Powers

There has been a rapidly increasing number of scientific discoveries in recent years related to foods of vegetable origin. As methods of chemical analysis have become more precise, it is being proved that fruits, grains, legumes and vegetables contain, in addition to nutrients found in all foods, two types of compounds that are *not found* in foods of **animal** origin:

- *antioxidants* (certain vitamins and minerals), and
- *phytochemicals* with curative properties.

Many scientists are inquisitive about the origin and significance of these beneficial substances found only in vegetables. *Why do humans need them for their health? Why do they continue to need them after centuries or millennia of adaptation to a carnivorous diet, such as the traditional diet of the Eskimos? Why is there an **ideal diet** for the health of humans?*

Two Options...

There are those that believe that humans found plants and vegetable foods possessing healing powers by mere chance. These vegetables, according to this reasoning, evolved the capacity to synthesize precisely those nutritional and healing substances that would be needed by humans long before humans existed.[4]

But we may also consider, with no less validity, a rational alternative:, that a superior Being created Man and Woman and provided them with an ideal "fuel": vegetable foods.[5]

Without a doubt many things have happened since then. Therefore in the present state of nature and humanity, **foods of animal origin** can become **necessary** *in some cases;* although *never* **indispensable.** This notwithstanding, the basis of human nutrition as well as the most important source of health-producing materials continue to be fruit, grains, seeds, and vegetables. The exception, of course, is the first phase of life (lactation).

...and the Same Conclusion

In either of these cases, no matter what one may believe about origins, numerous scientific studies demonstrate that vegetable foods prepared simply provide the *best* 'fuel' for our "engine." They supply the energy necessary to function and the substances to slow the "wear and tear" of the years and helps prevent "breakdown."

And do not forget to provide the *best* **oil** for this "engine!" (see p. 32).

Foods and Health

Our health depends on the sum total of the many **"small" decisions** that we take each day, in other words, our **lifestyle.**

Generally speaking, the decisions we make that *most affect* our health have to do with the **foods** we eat. There are so many options available that we must continually decide which foods to select and how they are best prepared.

Information + Correct Choices = Health

The more complete the information we have concerning available foods, the easier it is to make the best choices for health.[6]

Harmful Foods, Beneficial Foods

Humans need food throughout their lives. While all foods provide nutrients and energy, some can cause disorders and diseases; while others, bring health and healing. Therefore, there are potentially harmful foods, and, of course, beneficial foods.

(see p. 32).

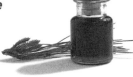

Foods of Animal Origin With Healing Properties

Although foods of vegetable origin hold the most healing powers, some of animal origin stand out because of their preventive and healing properties.

Honey and Other Products of the Hive

*Honey is referred to as **sweet medicine.** Royal jelly, pollen, and propolis act as a general tonic.*

Yogurt

Yogurt increases immune defenses because of the bacteria it contains, rather than because of its milk content.

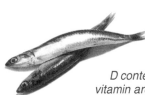

Fish

*Fish oils are used for their **anti-inflammatory** and **hypolipidemic** (lowers blood triglyceride levels) effects. Fish liver oil has long been used for the prevention and treatment of rickets because of its high vitamin D content although manufactured preparations of this vitamin are preferred today.*

Beef Liver

*Beef liver and that of other mammals has been used in the treatment of different types of **anemia,** because of its high content of iron and vitamin B_{12}. Manufactured products are preferred today, due, among other reasons, to the high level of chemical contamination present in the organs of animals.*

Throughout the pages that follow the reader will come to understand that all foods are not of equal value.

Knowing Foods Well

It is vital to understand foods well in order to select those that maintain our health, which is so threatened today, and those that treat various diseases. This magabook is designed to provide that understanding.

Foods can prevent and cure diseases, but they can also cause them. Therefore, the best diet is not one that includes "a little of everything" but one that avoids the harmful and makes moderate use of the beneficial.

Sources of Foods

Humans can adapt to eating almost anything, whether mineral, vegetable or animal. But simply because something can be eaten does not mean that this may be done without risking good health.

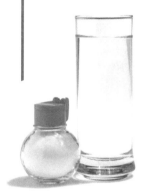

From the Mineral Kingdom

Water and **salt** are two foods (in the broad sense of the word), of mineral origin. Unlike any other food, the water and salt we eat do not originate with any living thing.

From the Animal Kingdom

Certain secretions, eggs, and meat of various aquatic and land animals can be used for food. However, ***not all*** of them are **beneficial.**

- The **milk** of various species of mammals and the dairy products that are made from it.

- **Honey** and other **secretions** of certain insects such as **bees.**

From the Vegetable Kingdom

These foods are the ***healthiest*** and have the ***most healing properties.*** Various types of vegetables can be used as food:

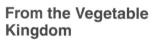

- **Seaweed:** These are eaten whole, whether they are microscopic single-cell (such as Spirulina) or multicellular such as the rest of the seaweed.

- **Higher plants:** Customarily, these foods are a part of the plant: fruit, seed, bulb, root, etc.

- **Fungi:** Although they are grouped with foods of vegetable origin, fungi belong to an independent kingdom with its own characteristics. Those fungi used as food are:

  - certain **microscopic** fungi belonging to the class Ascomycetes, such as brewer's yeast.
  - **mushrooms,** which are, in reality only a part (fruity body) of higher fungi.

- The **eggs** of some birds, especially those belonging to the family *Gallinaceae.*

- The **eggs** of certain **fish** such as the sturgeon (caviar).

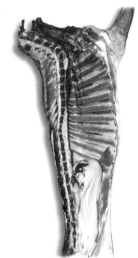

- The meat of a variety of **fish, mollusks, amphibians** and **crustaceans.**

- The **meat** and other body tissues of aquatic (whale) or land (lamb) **mammals.**

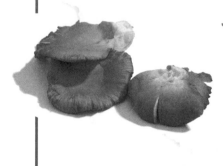

Comparison of Foods of Vegetable and Animal Origin

	Vegetable Origin	Animal Origin
Healing	***Yes.*** In addition to their nutritive properties, they act pharmacologically in a manner *similar* to **medicinal plants** (see next page).	Only ***very few*** and only in very specific cases.
Living	The greater portion can be eaten while their cells are still alive, therefore retaining ***all*** of their **biochemical and healing potential.**	Their cells are dead when eaten. **Decay** begins in these cells at the moment of the animal's death.
Chemical contamination	Generally speaking, this is ***very small and external.*** As a result peeling or thorough washing *can eliminate it.*	***Greater*** than with vegetables, since animals **retain and concentrate** contaminants that they consume.
Harmful components	Generally, they contain ***few and of low*** **toxicity.** Any that may be present are normally removed by soaking or cooking.	May contain very **powerful and dangerous toxins,** particularly seafood and some fish.
Depletion of natural resources	Production requires ***few*** natural resources. Some crops, such as legumes, do not even require fertilizer.	***High.*** To gain ***one*** calorie of **animal-based** food, it is necessary to provide ***seven*** calories of **vegetable-based** feed to livestock or fowl.
Antioxidant action	Fruits, as well as vegetables, are ***rich*** in **powerful** antioxidants such as vitamins A, C, and E, selenium and flavonoids. They *prevent* **premature aging,** *avoid* cancer and *enhance* the **immune system.**	Contains ***only a trace*** of antioxidants.
Diuretic	***Promotes*** **elimination** of numerous **prejudicial substances** that are the by-products of **metabolism,** such as uric acid and urea. **Purifies** and **detoxifies** the blood and tissues.	***Do not act*** as a diuretic. To the contrary, meat, seafood and fish **add** waste material to the organism.
Na/K quotient (sodium/potassium)	***Low,*** since they contain much more potassium than sodium. This *contributes* to its **diuretic** and **antihypertensive** effects.	***High.*** Dairy products, fish, seafood, and meats contain more sodium and less potassium than vegetables. Their ***regular consumption*** *may lead* to **hypertension.**
Ca/P quotient (calcium/phosphorous)	***High,*** thus *contributing* to the fixation of **minerals** in the **bones.**	***Low.*** Since they contain much more phosphorous than calcium fish, seafood, and meat act as **decalcifiers.**
Cholesterol	***No vegetable*** food contains cholesterol; not even those rich in fats such as nuts. Additionally they *help* **lower** blood cholesterol levels.	Cholesterol is ***only*** found in **foods of animal origin. All** animal secretions and animal tissues with the exception of honey and other products of the beehive contain cholesterol.
Heart	***Heart healthy,*** help *avoid* **arteriosclerosis.**	Milk products, eggs and meat are associated with **coronary disease.**
Cancer	Contain substances that ***counteract*** the effect of **carcinogens** consumed as ingredients of other foods or as a consequence of environmental pollution. Additionally, they *stop* the **development** of **cancerous cells.**	Several research studies relate the ***liberal use*** of milk, eggs and meat with various types of cancer. On the other hand, **yogurt** and **fermented milk** products have a ***prophylactic*** effect.

The Healing Power

Discover the natural pharmacy in your pantry.
This chart presents some of the healing properties of vegetable foods.

Celery

Diuretics

Celery: increases urine production, aids kidney function and reduces edema.

Other diuretic foods: eggplant, melon, watermelon, leeks, and asparagus.

Healing Foods

Plant-based foods, like medicinal plants, contain substances that produce pharmacological effects similar to any other medication, but with these **advantages:**

• They **prevent** and **correct the tendency toward** disease, in addition to having curative properties.

• *Generally* speaking, they *have no* **side effects.**

Astringents

Persimmon: Contains tannins that dry the intestinal mucosa and mucilage that softens it.

Other astringent foods: quince, apple, caimito, pomegranate, and loquat.

Persimmon

Hepatic Tonic

Artichoke

Artichoke: increases bile flow and detoxifies the liver.

Other foods that act as hepatic tonics: loquats, cardoom.

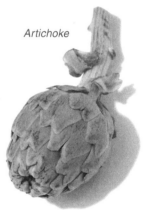

Urinary Antiseptics

Cranberry: Counters the effects of cystitis and other urinary infections without activating bacterial resistance.

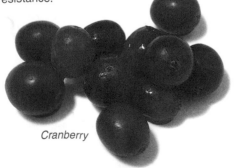
Cranberry

Mineral Restorers

Coconut: very rich in magnesium, calcium and phosphorous.

Other mineral restoring foods: almonds, alfalfa, cabbage, oranges, turnip greens.

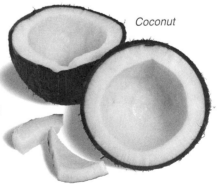
Coconut

# of Vegetables

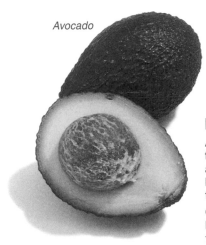

Avocado

Oranges

Hypolipidemic

Avocado: antianemic, protects the digestive lining and acts as a tonic in addition to lowering blood cholesterol and triglyceride levels.

Other hypolipidemic foods: beans, English walnuts, sunflower seeds, yams.

Antioxidants

Oranges: contain four potent antioxidants: vitamin C, beta-carotene (provitamin A), flavonoids and folic acid. They help avoid arteriosclerosis and thrombosis.

Other antioxidant foods: strawberries, citrus fruits, and nuts.

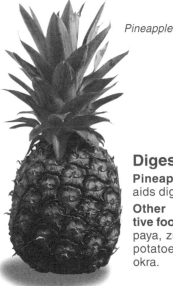

Pineapple

Anticarcinogens

Broccoli: Its phytochemicals retard or stop the growth of cancerous cells.

Other anticarcinogenic foods: Cauliflower, cabbage, oranges, lemons, plums, grapes, tomatoes.

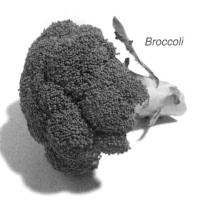

Broccoli

Digestives

Pineapple: aids digestion.

Other digestive foods: papaya, zucchini, potatoes, and okra.

Antianemics

Pistachios: Contain as much or more iron as lentils, in addition to copper and other trace elements that serve to promote blood production.

Other antianemic foods: red beets, apricots, passion fruit, spinach, and lamb's lettuce.

Laxatives

Plums: stimulate intestinal function.

Other laxative foods: eggplant, chard, and whole grain cereals.

Plums

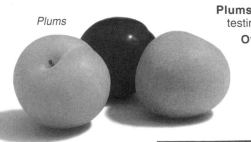

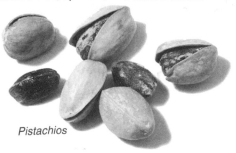

Pistachios

Exotic Fruits:

Fruits considered exotic in countries where they are not produced are just as healthful and nutritious as any other fruit. They do not possess any special properties not found in more common fruits, as was once thought. However, eating them gives a special pleasure that enriches the food experience. This chart displays some of the more attractive.

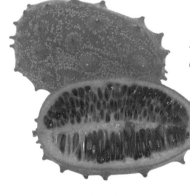

Kiwano

This native of Africa is, in reality, a wild cucumber, very aromatic and flavorful. The spines on its rind are fleshy and its pulp, gelatinous. It has **digestive** and **laxative** properties.

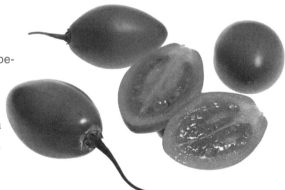

Tamarillo

Also called **tree tomato,** because of its appearance, which is similar to the tomato. They are native to South America. They are eaten fresh and have a slightly acid taste.

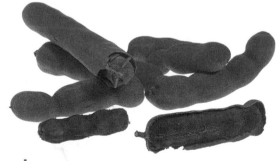

Tamarind

The slightly acid pulp of this legume-like fruit is an effective **laxative**.

Mangosteen

These are native of Thailand, where they are considered a true delicacy. Its bittersweet taste is reminiscent of plums.

Delights of Paradise

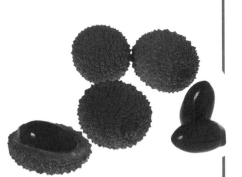

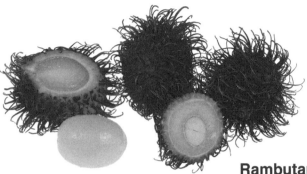

Rambutan

This native of Malaysia has a pulp similar to the litchi, with a flavor similar to almonds.

Litchi

This fruit of a tree from China is noted for its **high vitamin C content,** which is greater than that of oranges or lemons. They enhance the **immune system**.

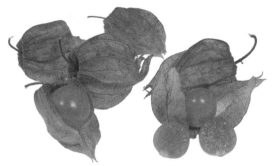

Winter Cherry

Originating in East Asia and China, these are now grown in Colombia. It is like a cherry with a pleasantly tart flavor.

Attracted by the Exotic

In European countries, particularly, **'exotic'** fruits are those coming from faraway, generally tropical, places. Their brilliant colors, unique shapes, and delicate aromas have always attracted travelers and explorers. Today, thanks to better transport, more and more exotic fruits are finding their way to the markets of the world.

Two historic figures stand out as special contributors to our knowledge of tropical fruits:

Christopher Columbus was so taken by the richness of the vegetation in Central America that he thought he had found the earthly Paradise. He and his men brought many American species to Spain, thus making them known for the first time in Europe in the 16th century.

Georg Meister, a German botanist, traveled to Southeast Asia in the 17th century in search of new fruits. Ten years later, never ceasing to marvel at the "magnificent work of the Eternal in these beautiful lands", he returned to his native Saxony. In 1692 he published an illustrated book on exotic fruits that constitutes one of the great classics of universal botany.

Many fruits ceased being exotic when they acclimatized and were cultivated in other places. For example, the orange was considered exotic in 15th century Europe when it was introduced to the West from China. The same has happened with the avocado and cherimoya, which have been successfully grown in southern Spain for many years.

Night-Blooming Cereus

This fruit is covered with spines, like the cactus that it is. Its pulp, however, is very sweet and aromatic.

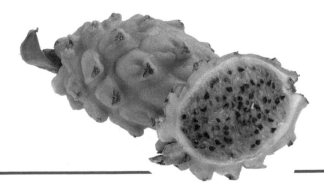

Nutritional Value

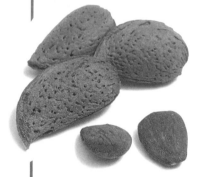
Almonds

Nuts Provide:

- *Energy:* Of all natural foods, nuts provide the *most* **calories** in proportion to weight.

- *Fats:* Approximately *half* of their **weight** is liquid fat (oil) that is *very rich* in **mono and polyunsaturated fatty acids** (except the coconut whose fats are predominantly saturated). **Walnuts** are particularly rich in linolenic acid, a precursor of the **omega-3** fatty acids.
  As a result, nuts *reduce* LDL **cholesterol (harmful),** *increase* **HDL cholesterol** (beneficial), and protect against **arteriosclerosis.**

- *Protein:* Nuts follow only **legumes** in protein content. Their protein content is usually *greater than* **meat, fish, eggs, and grains.**
  The proteins in nuts are *quite* **complete,** being deficient only in the amino acids lysine and methionine. They are well supplemented by **legumes** (rich in lysine) and **grains** (rich in methionine), as well as **milk.**

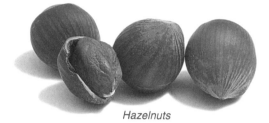
Hazelnuts

- *Minerals:* The **almond** is the nut *richest* in **calcium. Pistachios and peanuts** provide the *most* **iron.**[7] **Sesame and sunflower seeds** have even *more* **iron** than nuts. Both seeds and nuts have *very high* levels of **magnesium** and **phosphorus.**

- *Vitamins:* Nuts are a *good source* of vitamins B_1, B_2, B_6, E, pantothenic acid, and folates. About 75% of the vitamin B_1 is destroyed in the roasting process.
  Nuts are a *good source* of **choline,** a vitamin factor that forms part of lecithin, and improves liver function.

- *Trace elements:* Nuts are *very rich* in zinc, manganese, copper, and selenium.

- *Phytochemicals:* Nuts contain many substances that are very active throughout the organism:
  - *Ellagic acid, flavonoids,* and **phenolic compounds,** all of which are potent **antioxidants;**
  - *Phytosterols:* substances similar to cholesterol but of vegetable origin, that *block the absorption* of **cholesterol** in the intestine;
  - *Isoflavons:* similar to those contained in soy, but in lower proportions. Isoflavons *protect against* **arteriosclerosis, osteoporosis, and cancer.**

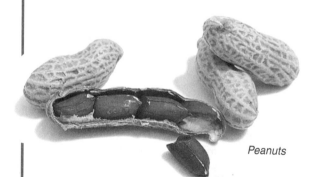
Peanuts

Portion of Some Nutrients per 100 g of Nuts

Nut	Calories	Carbohydrates	Fats	Protein	Vitamin E	Calcium	Iron	Fiber
ALMONDS	586 kcal	11.8 g	52.5 g	20.4 g	20.3 mg α-TE	247 mg	3.63 mg	6.7 g
HAZELNUTS	632 kcal	9.2 g	62.6 g	13 g	23.9 mg α-TE	188 mg	3.27 mg	6.1 g
PEANUTS	567 kcal	7.64 g	49.2 g	25.8 g	9.13 mg α-TE	92 mg	4.58 mg	8.5 g
WALNUTS	642 kcal	13.5 g	61.9 g	14.3 g	2.62 mg α-TE	94 mg	2.44 mg	4.8 g

# of Nuts

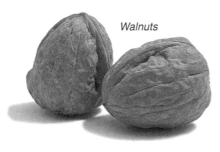
Walnuts

Nuts Do Not Contain:

- *provitamin A,* nor
- *vitamin C*

Fresh **fruits** and **vegetables** *compensate* for these vitamin deficiencies.

 Benefits of Nuts

- They provide **energy** and are *very* **nutritious.**
- They can be eaten **raw,** as nature intended, without need for further processing.
- They are a *healthful* **alternative** to **meat** given their richness in protein, minerals, and vitamins.
- In addition to containing *no* **cholesterol,** they are *effective* **in reducing** blood cholesterol levels.[8,9,10]
- They *protect* the **heart's health** by reducing the risk of coronary heart disease, such as **heart attack** and **angina pectoris.** This has shown to be the case in persons that eat nuts in place of other fatty foods.
- They *do not* **cause obesity.** To the contrary, they aid weight loss when nuts replace other high-calorie foods in the diet. **Calorie for calorie, they are** *less* **fattening** than high-fat foods such as sausages, aged cheeses, sweets, and pastries or ice cream.
- Due to their very low carbohydrate level, they are *well tolerated* by **diabetics.**[11]
- They *do not* **produce uric acid.**

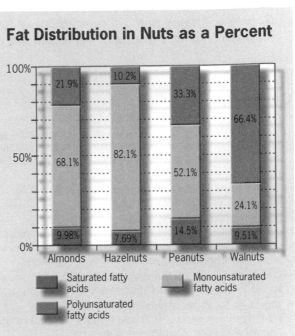

Fat Distribution in Nuts as a Percent

	Almonds	Hazelnuts	Peanuts	Walnuts
Polyunsaturated	21.9%	10.2%	33.3%	66.4%
Monounsaturated	68.1%	82.1%	52.1%	24.1%
Saturated	9.98%	7.69%	14.5%	9.51%

■ Saturated fatty acids   ■ Monounsaturated fatty acids

■ Polyunsaturated fatty acids

The higher the mono and polyunsaturated fatty acid levels, the greater the beneficial effect on cholesterol level.

Drawbacks to Nuts

- They must be well chewed. Whole nuts may present difficulty for children and the elderly, who may eat them either in paste or creme.
- They may produce **indigestion** in persons with digestive system disorders. To improve tolerance they should be:
  - eaten raw or lightly roasted (not fried),
  - limited to eating no more than 50 g (about 2 ounces) at one time,
  - chewed well or ground, and the skin should be removed by blanching in scalding hot water.
- They may cause **allergenic reactions** in small children and should not be given to infants under the age of 12 months. In any case they should be introduced gradually. The **pine nut** or piñon nut is the *best tolerated* **by small children.**

Nutritional value

Some see grains and grain products as foods that only provide carbohydrates and calories. However, whole grains in particular are a good source of protein, minerals and vitamins.

Grains Provide:

- *Digestible carbohydrates* (50%-60% of grain weight): Most is in the form of *starch,* which is converted to *glucose* by digestive **enzymes**. The glucose is then absorbed into the blood through the small intestine and provides **energy** to the entire body.

- *Indigestible carbohydrates (cellulose fiber):* particularly in **whole grains** and their products.

- *Protein* (7.5%-17% of grain weight): Grain proteins are of a *sufficient quality* to meet the needs of **adults. Children,** on the other hand, need to *supplement* grain products with other *lysine-rich* foods such as **milk** or **legumes.**

- **Oats and wheat** are the *most* protein-rich grains in relation to their caloric content; **corn and rice** are the least.

- *Vitamins B₁, B₂, B₆, E, niacin and folates:* are found particularly in the **germ** and **bran.** This means that **refined** grains have *very little* of these nutrients.

- *Minerals and trace elements:* **whole-grain** products contain *much more* phosphorous, magnesium, iron, calcium, zinc, and selenium than those that are more refined.

- *Phytochemical elements:* lignans, phytoestrogens (similar to the isoflavons found in soy), phytic acid and phytates and phenolic compounds that act as **antioxidants.**[13]

Grains *Do Not* Contain:

- *Provitamin A* (except corn),

- *vitamin C,*

- *vitamin B₁₂,*

On the other hand, **sprouts** from grain do contain *provitamin A* and *vitamin C.* As mentioned, these vitamins are missing in dried grains.

Grain: a Complete Unit

All grains are made up of three components: **bran, endosperm and germ**.

According to the principles of Dr. *Bircher-Benner,* these three components form a complete unit whose nutritional value surpasses the nutritional value of the bran, endosperm or germ separately.

It is *wisest* to eat the **whole grain** just as it is provided by nature, since it contains the *ideal* **proportion of nutrients.**

❶ **Bran:** rich in fiber, vitamins and minerals. The *most widely used* brans are that of **wheat** for its laxative action, and those of **oats** for its **cholesterol** *lowering properties.*[12] Bran from barley, rice, and corn are also used.

❷ **Endosperm or nucleus:** Formed by granules of starch and proteins.

❸ **Germ:** *very rich en B vitamins* and *vitamin E.* **Wheat germ** is the most used.

Proteins

Fiber

Starch

Minerals

Vitamins

Fat

# of Grains

Benefits of Grains
(particularly whole grains)

- **They contain *more nutrients*** than refined products, particularly more vitamins and minerals. *Eating **whole-grain products*** has ***no adverse effect on the absorption** of minerals.*[16] As a result; those suffering from iron deficiency anemia can safely use them. The use of ***bran alone*** **reduce absorption of *iron*** and ***zinc.***
- **They are *rich*** in ***fiber:*** This insoluble cellulose fiber that acts like a "broom" sweeping the digestive tract.
- **They produce a greater sense of satiety** because of their fiber content. The fiber swells in the stomach. This *helps* reduce additional food intake, thus *preventing* **obesity.**
- **They help avoid constipation:** eating whole grains improves intestinal function:[17]
  - Increases fecal volume
  - Accelerates fecal passage through the intestines
  - Facilitates the elimination of toxic substances, such as bile acids.
- **They reduce cancer risk,** especially that of the colon[18] and the breast, when whole-grains are eaten regularly.
- **They help avoid coronary disease and arteriosclerosis:** The protective effects of whole grains regarding cardiovascular disease[19] are due to high levels of:
  - ***antioxidants***[20] (vitamin E, selenium, phenolic compounds, etc.),
  - ***unsaturated fatty acids*** (in the germ),
  - ***trace elements,***
  - ***phytochemicals*** (lignans, phytoestrogens),
  - cellulose ***fiber.***
- **They prevent diabetes:** A study conducted at Harvard University (USA) demonstrated that the more whole-grain products eaten, the lower the risk of non-insulin dependent diabetes.[21]
  Because the glucose in whole grains is released slowly, it does not produce abrupt increases in its blood level. As a result, diabetics **tolerate whole-grain products *better* than those of refined grains,** and can eat them without difficulty.
- **They do not contain cholesterol,** and contribute to the reduction of its level in the blood.

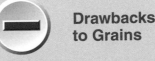

Drawbacks to Grains

- **Their proteins are deficient in lysine.** This deficit can be made up in two ways:
  - *Combining* them *with* **milk** or **legumes.**
  - Eating **varieties of grains** that have been genetically engineered to contain *high levels of lysine.* Since their protein is complete, they are *ideal* for **infant diets.** The problem with these hybrids is that they yield 10% to 15% less per planted area, and are therefore more expensive.
- They **acidify** the blood and the internal organs to some extent, but to a much lesser extent than cheese, meat or fish.
- **Its abuse may cause malnutrition:** Eating *excessive* quantities of grain products satisfies the appetite. While this may supply protein and calorie needs, *other foods* containing necessary nutrients *are neglected.* This can occur when infants are overfed with cereals. This creates a condition known as **farinaceous dystrophy.**
- **Contraindicated in cases of celiac disease** (gluten intolerance). *Only* **rice** and **corn** contain *no gluten* and can be safely eaten by those suffering from this disorder.
- **Allergies:** Some children with atopic eczemas and other symptoms of skin allergies improve when gluten is removed from their diet.[14]
- **Anti-nutritive factors:** Whole grain bran contain **phytates** that can interfere with the absorption of various minerals such as iron and zinc.
  However, *soaking, fermenting* (through the natural leavening process of breadmaking), and *sprouting* of the grain virtually *eliminate* its **phytate** content[15] as well as other **anti-nutritive factors** that may be present in the bran.

Composition of Pasta

Necessary ingredients:

- **Semolina made from hard wheat:** hard wheat contains more gluten than soft or common wheat. This results in pasta with better consistency. Semolina from soft wheat can be used but it requires that an egg be added to the dough.

- **Water.**

Optional ingredients:

- **Egg:** gives more consistency to the pasta and makes it more nutritious. In some countries eggs are required for making noodles.

- **Vegetables:** These are blended to a paste or puree and added to the dough. They add vitamins, minerals and a touch of color. The most used vegetables are spinach, carrots, artichokes, and tomato.

- **Protein supplements,** such as soy flour, non-fat powdered milk or wheat gluten. Pastas that are prepared in this way are described as **fortified.**

- **Vitamin and mineral supplements:** Pastas that have these added are called **enriched** (see the next page). These supplements may be:
  - *artificial:* iron and B group vitamins, or
  - *natural:* brewer's yeast, torula yeast, wheat germ.

Making Pasta

Although in many parts of Italy pasta making is done by hand, the usual industrial method consists of the following steps:

1. **Prepare semolina:** After soaking hard wheat to make bran removal easier, the grain is coarsely ground to a specific particle size. This, and not flour, is ideal for making pasta.

2. **Preparation of the dough:** Even though the main ingredient is semolina, some flour is usually added. The dough must not ferment. To avoid the formation of bubbles that would weaken the pasta, the dough is placed in a mechanical vacuum.

3. **Extrusion of the pasta,** which consists of forcing the dough under pressure through molds that give it the desired shape.

4. **Drying** and hardening. **Fresh pasta** pasta is sold without drying, but it cannot be stored as long as dry.

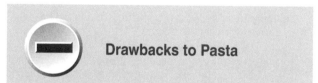

Drawbacks to Pasta

- Made from **refined grain:** Even though whole-grain pasta is available, it is generally made of refined wheat semolina that has had the bulk of the bran and germ removed. Therefore, as is the case with white bread, it is lacking in *fiber, B vitamins,* and *minerals.* This issue can be *compensated* for by:

  - **Enriching it** it with minerals and vitamins (generally iron, vitamins B_1 and B_2 and niacin). This only compensates for the loss of a few nutrients lost in the refining process.
  - Adding **brewer's or torula yeast** and/or **wheat germ,** as is done by some commercial manufacturers. This is a *better approach* than enrichment since all of these products are rich in vitamins, minerals and trace elements.
  - Eating it *with* **vegetables.**

- **Its protein is deficient in lysine,** as is the case with all grains and their derivatives. This can be partially compensated for by *fortifying* it with egg or soy flour.

- It may *exacerbate* symptoms of **flatulence, acidification of the blood** and **celiac disease** and should be avoided by persons suffering from these conditions.

Benefits of Pasta

- **It stores easily** without need for refrigeration, except fresh pasta.

- **It is easy to cook.**

- Its **neutral flavor** allows it to be easily combined with a wide variety of sauces and other complements.

- It is **easily digested** and well tolerated by those with digestive difficulties.

- It is *rich* in **carbohydrates and protein,** but *low* in **fats,** which helps compensate for the fats present in the typical Western diet.

- It provides *sufficient* **calories,** which makes it an **excellent food** for **children, those active in sports and active people in general.**

All Shapes

Types of Pasta

Italy, and Naples in particular, seems to be the birth-place of pasta. From there it has extended throughout the world. More than 300 kinds of pasta are made in its native land. These can be grouped in five types:

- **Dry:** 100g are more than enough for an adult. For example, 100 g of maca-roni provide 72.3 g car-bohydrates, 12.8 g protein, 1.6 g fat, 2.4 g fiber and 371 kcal.

- **Enriched and/or fortified:** adding egg, soy flour, brewer's yeast, wheat germ, or vegetables increases its nutritional value.

- **Whole-grain:** This is the richest in fiber, vitamins, and minerals.

- **Filled:** This consists of laminated dough filled with various products such as cheese, meat, spinach, etc. *Ravioli* and *tortellini* are the best known.

- **Fresh:** Since it has not been dried, it has a soft texture, which makes it easier to prepare, and takes less time to cook. But it can only be stored for a few days.

The Secret to Perfect Pasta

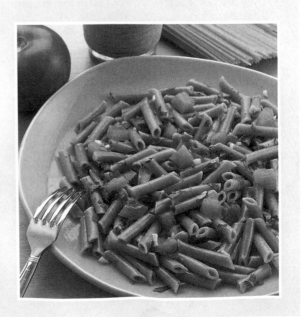

1. Place an appropriate, uncovered kettle on the stove with *one liter* (about 4 cups) **of water** for each *100 g* (about 4 ounces) **of pasta.**

2. Heat the water **to a boil. Add the pasta a *small amount at a time*** so the water does not stop boiling. Add about *6 g* (about 1 teaspoon) **of salt** for each liter of water. Stir occasionally with a wooden spoon to prevent sticking.

3. Fresh pasta requires only 3 or 4 minutes of cooking.

4. Dry pasta should be removed from the heat when it is *al dente;* in other words, well cooked but firm in consistency.

5. **Drain** in a colander *without* rinsing with **cold water.**

6. After draining, add a little oil to keep the pasta from sticking.

*Persons who cannot tolerate cooked legumes can,
however, eat their sprouts, which are germinated seeds.*

Changes that Take Place During Sprouting

When a seed has the water, oxygen, and heat necessary, it begins to sprout to form a new living thing, a new plant, which will in time produce more seeds. Sprouting begins with numerous chemical processes facilitated by enzymes. Thanks to this the following changes in the seed take place:

Benefits of Sprouts

- **They are living foods:** Even though fruit, grain, and vegetables are living foods in their natural condition, in sprouts **life** is present *with all* of its **vigor.** This means that sprouts are *rich* in substances that are of *great* **biological** *value* necessary for our bodies, such as *vitamins* and *enzymes.*

- **They are predigested:** the enzymes that are synthesized during the sprouting process *begin* the **digestion** of *starch, protein,* and *fats* that are in the seeds. This chemical process is similar to what takes place in the body during digestion. For this reason, sprouts are *easy* to **digest** and are **assimilated** *very well.*
  They contain *many* **nutrients** and proportionately *few* **calories,** which makes them useful in diets against obesity.

- **They have medicinal properties:**
  – They stimulate the digestive process.
  – They regenerate intestinal flora.
  – They are antioxidants, depurative and mineralizing.

- **They are simple to prepare** and may be eaten just as they are raw in salads or in a variety of cooked dishes.

- **They make us aware** of the value of natural life processes. Watching the sprouting of a simple seed makes us appreciate more how extraordinary the phenomena of life are.

- **Transformation** of reserve substances;
  – Large **starch** molecules are broken into smaller ones, such as **dextrin** and **maltose,** which will be converted into **glucose** in the digestive system.
  – The **proteins** are transformed into fragments with smaller numbers of **amino acids** (peptides) and **free amino acids.**
  – The *fats release* the **fatty acids** of which they are composed.

- **Synthesis** of new substances, such as:
  – **vitamin C,** which was not present in the seed;
  – **chlorophyll,** which is very healthful.

- **Elimination of antinutritional factors** that are found in the seed, particularly in legumes, such as **hemaglutinin, phytic acid, and protease inhibitors**. It is necessary to cook legumes to deactivate these substances, but they **disappear** with **sprouting.**

Sprouting Technique

Although sprouts are available commercially, it is an interesting experience growing them at home following the following steps:

1. Use only seeds intended for domestic sprouting. **Seeds** destined for **agricultural use** may be treated with **pesticides** or other **chemical products.**

2. Put the seeds to soak in a glass (*never in metal*) container covered with a fine cloth such as cheesecloth. The amount of water should be three or four times the volume of the seeds.

3. Place the container in a **warm, dark place for about 12 hours.**

4. After 12 hours, discard the water and **rinse the seeds with *tepid* water.** After that, **rinse the seeds and change the water *two or three times* a day** until they sprout (this usually takes 2 to 5 days).

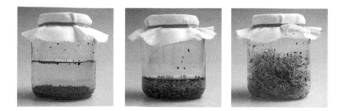

Living Foods

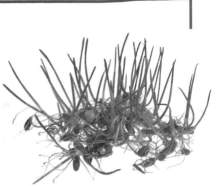

The Most Valued Sprouts:

Any legume or grain seed can be sprouted, however, the most valued for their tenderness and flavor are those obtained from:

- Legumes:
  - **mung bean** (also known as green gram),
  - **alfalfa**.
- Grains:
  - wheat
  - barley

It is also possible to sprout seeds of watercress, radish, pumpkin, sunflower, flax, sesame, etcetera.

Possible Drawbacks to Sprouts

- **Toxic:** *Raw* legumes contain toxic *antinutritional factors,* such as hemaglutinin. For this reason they must *always be cooked.* Sprouting with appropriate soaking, as has been described, removes these toxic substances entirely.[22, 23, 24]
  Alfalfa sprouts contain a small amount of a non-protein amino acid (l-canavanine), which can produce toxic effects to those suffering of erythematous lupus.

- *Phytates:* Raw legumes and grains contain phytates, which have, in spite of being anticarcinogens, the undesirable effect of *interfering* with the **absorption** of *iron, calcium,* and *zinc.* However, during **sprouting**, these *disappear* for the most part.[25]

- *Saponins:* These substances found in seeds, *increase* during the sprouting process. Saponins were found to destroy red blood cells in *in vitro* laboratory experiments. For this reason they were considered toxic. However, today it has been proved that *in vivo,* that is, in the human body, they do not produce hemolysis (the destruction of blood cells). To the contrary, *saponins* are *beneficial,* since:
  - They *reduce* the level of blood **cholesterol,**[26, 27]
  - they are **anticarcinogens**.[28]

- **Bacterial contamination:** There have been cases of alfalfa seeds and sprouts contaminated with the bacteria *Salmonella stanley.*[29] Treatment with chlorinated antiseptics can reduce the number of bacteria, but do not eliminate them completely.[30, 31] It is advisable to use sprouts from a reliable and hygienic source.

MUNG BEAN, SPROUTED
Composition
per 100 g of raw edible portion

Energy	30.0 kcal = 126 kj
Protein	3.04 g
Carbohydrates	4.13 g
Fiber	1.80 g
Vitamin A	2.00 µg RE
Vitamin B₁	0.084 mg
Vitamin B₂	0.124 mg
Niacin	1.37 mg NE
Vitamin B₆	0.088 mg
Folate	60.8 µg
Vitamin B₁₂	—
Vitamin C	13.2 mg
Vitamin E	0.010 mg α-TE
Calcium	13.0 mg
Phosphorus	54.0 mg
Magnesium	21.0 mg
Iron	0.910 mg
Potassium	149 mg
Zinc	0.410 mg
Total Fat	0.180 g
Saturated Fat	0.046 g
Cholesterol	—
Sodium	6.00 mg

1% 2% 4% 10% 20% 40% 100%

% Daily Value (based on a 2,000 calorie diet)
provided by 100 g of this food

PERCENTAGE COMPOSITION

Fiber **1.80 %**
Minerals **0.440 %**
Carbohydr. **4.13 %**
Fat **0.180 %**
Protein **3.04 %**
Water **90.4 %**

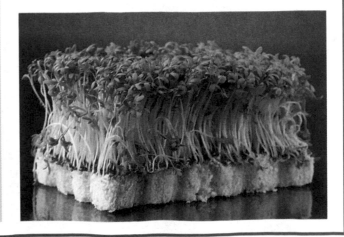

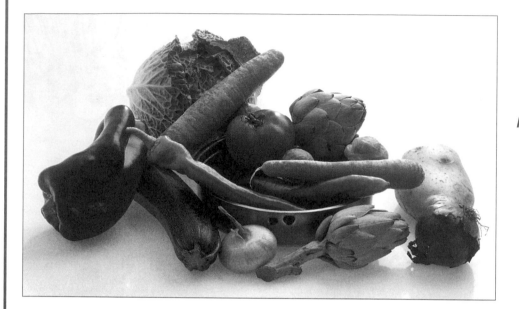

Stalks

These, such as **asparagus** and **leeks,** are *rich* in *fiber* and are generally **diuretic. Sugar** cane is a stalk that stores great quantities of a type of sugar called sucrose.

In some cases only parts of some stalks, called shoots, are eaten. Examples are **bamboo shoots** and palm **hearts.**

Leeks

Leaves

These are more nutritious than one might believe. The leaves of **turnips, parsnips,** and **cabbage** are good sources of *calcium.* **Spinach** is a good source of *iron.* They also contain between 1% and 3% *protein.*

Some leaves, such as **spinach** and **sorrel** contain *oxalic acid* that can interfere with the absorption of calcium.

Cabbage leaves contain **anti-carcinogenic phytochemicals**.

Brussels Sprouts

Flowers and Buds

Artichokes, cauliflower, and **broccoli** are inflorescent vegetables, meaning that they are made up of tightly bunched florets. They contain *provitamin A* as well as *vitamins B and C.*

Artichokes

Vegetables

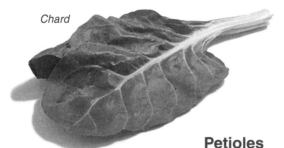

Chard

Petioles

These are the stems connecting the leaves to the stalk. In some plants, such as **cardoon** and **chard,** they are so developed that they become very tender and flavorful. Like stalks, petioles are rich in **cellulose.**

Seeds

Peas and **beans** are the seeds of plants of the *Leguminosae* family that are used as vegetables. As with all seeds, they are a *good source of protein.*

Beans

Tubers

These are not roots but rather specialized underground enlargements of the plant's stalk. They are the storage site for *starch,* which is the *primary* reserve substance in **vegetables.** They contain some level of *protein* as well as *vitamin C* (for example, the **potato**) and *provitamin A* **(sweet potato).**

Tubers should *not* be eaten *raw* since they contain **toxic substances,** which are removed by cooking.

Potatoes

Fruits

From the bright red of the **tomato,** the brilliant purple of the **eggplant,** the orange and yellow of **pumpkins** and **squash** to the varied greens of **cucumbers, zucchini,** and **avocado,** these vegetables are notable for their colors.

The **avocado** is a special fruit since it contains between 15% and 17% *fat.* We consider it a vegetable because of the way it is used, even though it comes from a tree rather than a herbaceous plant.

Cucumbers

Roots

These contain carbohydrates (**starch**), **fiber,** and **minerals.** Some, such as **carrots** and **red beets,** contain beta-carotene (**provitamin A**).

Carrots

Bulbs

Bulbs are an underground thickening of the stalk that is formed by numerous layers. They contain sulfurous (**onions, garlic**) or aromatic (**fennel**) substances.

Garlic

Nutritional Value

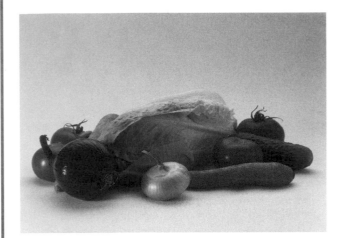

Even though the bulk of their weight is water, vegetables represent a veritable natural pharmacy of minerals, vitamins, and phytochemicals.

Vegetables Provide:

- *Water:* Most vegetables contain 90% to 95% water. This is even more than milk, which contains less than 88%. But this does not mean they are low in nutritional value. The remaining 5% to 10% of solids contain substances of great biological and therapeutic value.
- *Minerals:* Vegetables are a **good source** of *all* minerals. This explains their **alkalizing** effect and resulting benefit on the blood and tissues. The minerals most abundant in vegetables are:
  - *Potassium:* important for **diuretic and hypotensive** effect (lowers arterial blood pressure).
  - *Calcium:* Cabbage, for example, contains between 35 and 77 milligrams (mg) of calcium per 100 grams (g) of weight. This is a relatively important amount when compared with milk, which contains 119 mg per 100 g. Additionally; the body *easily* **absorbs** the *calcium* found in **cabbage.**[32]
  - *Iron:* **Spinach** contains 2.71 mg/100 g, which is more than the iron contained in **meat. Lamb's lettuce, fava beans, peas,** and **beets** are also good sources of iron. The *vitamin C* in these vegetables enhances the **absorption** of iron.
- *Vitamins:* in particular **provitamin A** (beta-carotene that is found in orange and red-colored vegetables), and *vitamins C, B* (except B_{12}), and *K* (found in alfalfa, cabbage, and spinach).

- *Folic acid and Folates:* These are **abundant** in *leafy green vegetables,* particularly in **spinach. Folic acid is an essential** nutrient for **pregnant women.**
- *Fiber:* Contributes to the feeling of satiation and satisfaction associated with eating. It also works to *prevent* **constipation.**
- *Proteins:* Vegetables contain significant amounts of protein that should not be overlooked. These proteins are generally superior to those found in fruits, although inferior to those in grains and legumes. Keeping in mind that a serving of vegetables may be as much as one cup, it becomes evident that such serving may provide a fair amount of proteins. For example, consider the milligrams of protein per 100 grams of some common vegetables: lettuce, 1.62; potatoes, 2.07; asparagus, 2.28; spinach, 2.86; Brussels sprouts, 3.38; peas, 5.42.

The proteins found in vegetables contain all of the essential and non-essential *amino acids* with two important considerations:

- Vegetables do not provide an adequate level of *methionine* to meet the body's need. However, **grains** are very *rich* in this essential amino acid.
- Vegetables contain *abundant lysine,* an essential amino acid that is found in very *low levels* in **grains.**

Vegetables and grains *together* provide **complete protein** thanks to the phenomenon of **supplementation. The protein** in **potatoes** is the **most complete** found in any vegetable.

- *Carbohydrates:* Only tubers such as the **potato** contain significant amounts.
- *Chlorophyll:* This is the green pigment found in all plants. While its effect in the body is not well known, it is thought to facilitate blood production.
- *Phytochemicals:* These constitute a very recent discovery in nutrition science. **Vegetables,** together with **fruit** and **legumes,** are the foods richest in these elements. Even though they are found only in very small amounts, they act as powerful **antioxidants** that help in the prevention of **cancer** and **coronary disease.**

The vegetables *richest* in these elements are those that belong to these two botanical families:

- **Cruciferae:** cabbage, radish, turnip, and watercress.
- **Liliaceae:** onions, garlic, and leeks.

The phytochemicals found in these two groups are rich in sulfur, which gives them their piquant taste.

# of Vegetables

Benefits of Vegetables

They are a Complement to Grains and Legumes

Vegetables provide nutrients that are lacking in the other two types of foods: *Pro-vitamin A, vitamin C,* and *folates.*

Beans

Natural Laxatives

The *fiber* content of vegetables increases the volume of fecal matter and facilitates its passage through the digestive tract. When vegetables are not tender, their fiber may be indigestible. In this case, they are best eaten grated or cooked.

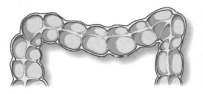

Ideal in Cases of Obesity

Maintain your weight by eating vegetables. They contain almost no *fat* and their **caloric content** is *very low.* However, they produce a sensation of satiation that substantially relieves feelings of hunger.

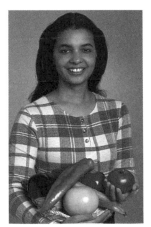

Appropriate For the Elderly

Because of their low caloric content, their **calcifying action,** and their **anti-carcinogenic** effect they are an excellent food for older persons.

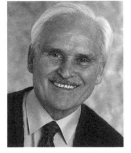

Source of Minerals

Turnip greens contain more *calcium* than **milk,** in addition to *magnesium, phosphorous,* and other minerals. **Cabbage** is also a good source of *calcium.* In general, stalks and leaves vegetables are rich in the *minerals* that build bone tissue. As such, they are recommended in cases of **osteoporosis** and other **calcium deficiency** disorders.

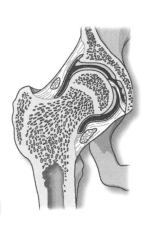

Diuretics and Antihypertensives

Because of their **potassium** content they *increase* urine production and *reduce* arterial **blood pressure.**

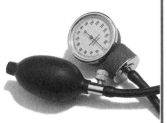

Antianemic

All vegetables, but particularly **beets, fava beans, spinach, watercress,** and **lamb's lettuce** *facilitate* the production of **red blood cells** due to their high **iron** content (whose absorption is facilitated by the simultaneous effect of *vitamin C* in the digestive system), as well as *trace elements* and *chlorophyll.*

Lamb's lettuce

Anticarcinogens

All vegetables, especially those of the family *Cruciferae* (**cabbage, radish, and turnip**) and *Liliaceae* (**onions, garlic, and leeks**) families, contain substances which have been shown to be *effective in vitro,* as well as *in vivo* to:

* *neutralize* the action of **carcinogenic substances** that promote cellular degeneration and,
  * *slow* the **growth** when the cancer process has already begun.

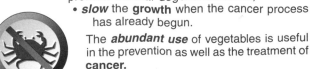

The *abundant use* of vegetables is useful in the prevention as well as the treatment of **cancer.**

Olive Oil:

Advantages of Olive oil Over Seed Oils

- **Ideal composition:** Main nutrients found in olive oil are:
  - triglycerides formed from glycerin and various fatty acids,
  - vitamin E: 12.4 mg α-TE/100 g and
  - iron: 0.38 mg/100 g

  Its distribution of fatty acids, with monounsaturated **oleic acid** prevailing, *comes the closest to the optimum* according to the American Heart Association, as can be seen in the graphs following graphs.

- **Better flavor:** The aroma and flavor of olive oil are more pronounced than those of seed oils, which are quite insipid. Although some persons are not used to the flavor of olive oil and prefer other oils with a neutral flavor, very few do not come to appreciate the *bouquet* of an excellent virgin olive oil.

- **More natural:** Its production process is simpler and more natural than that of seed oils. Virgin olive oil is **not refined** nor is it processed with **solvents**, as most seed oils are. Additionally, olive oil does not contain **trans-fatty acids.**

- **More stable:** Since it contains fewer **polyunsaturated fatty acids**, it is more stable than seed oils. It lasts longer before becoming rancid and producing dangerous **peroxides**.

- **Better for frying:** Resists **higher temperatures without decomposing**. For this reason, it is appropriate for frying.

- **Greater medical value:** A black legend has been about for quite some time in certain Anglo-Saxon regions suggesting that olive oil raises blood cholesterol.

Fortunately, **studies** regarding the Mediterranean diet *have demonstrated* that olive oil **protects the heart** *more* than any other, thus leading, on the whole, to the cardiac benefits of the Mediterranean diet.

Proportional Distribution of Different Types of Fatty Acids

*With the objective of preventing cardiac disease (angina and myocardial infarction), the American Heart Association (AHA)[134] recommends that **fats represent no more than 30%** of dietary calories. This percentage is less than that of the average Western diet, which averages 40% of its calories from fats.*

For a 2,000 calorie diet, the 30% is 600 calories; these are obtained from 67 g of fats (65 g to facilitate calculations).

Until the 1990s, the AHA recommended that these 67 grams of fats should be distributed in equal portions among saturated, monounsaturated and polyunsaturated.

However, in light of the latest studies, which highlight the importance of monounsaturated fatty acids, the AHA has modified the percentage distribution of the different fatty acids.

*Now the AHA says that rather than one third, fully **one half** of the daily intake of **fatty acids** should be **monounsaturated.** Olive oil and avocado are the healthier source of oleic acid, the main **monounsaturated** fatty acid of diet.*

These AHA recommendations coincide with those of the WHO (World Health Organization).[135]

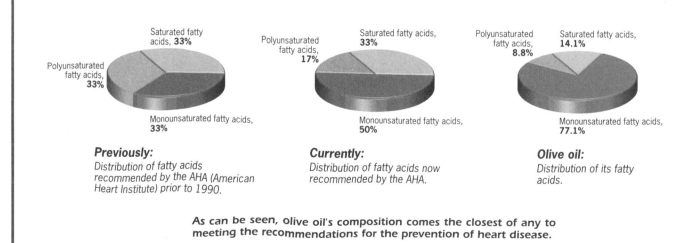

Previously:
Distribution of fatty acids recommended by the AHA (American Heart Institute) prior to 1990.

Currently:
Distribution of fatty acids now recommended by the AHA.

Olive oil:
Distribution of its fatty acids.

As can be seen, olive oil's composition comes the closest of any to meeting the recommendations for the prevention of heart disease.

the Ideal Formula

Olive oil is superior to seed oils as much for its dietary therapeutic properties, as for its flavor and aroma.

Medicinal Effects of Olive Oil

- **It promotes heart health.** Regular consumption of olive oil *protects* against coronary disease **(angina** and **myocardial infarction)**.

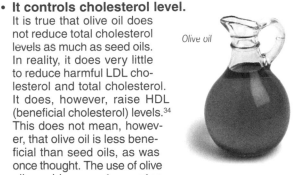

  - **It reduces the threat of thrombosis.** In a study in South Africa by the famous cardiac surgeon Christian Barnard, the first to perform a successful heart transplant, demonstrated that olive oil is *as effective* as fish oils in *reducing* the level of **fibrinogen** in the blood.[33] This protein substance is the primary component of blood clots; the higher its level, the greater the threat of **thrombosis** (formation of clots).

- **It controls cholesterol level.** It is true that olive oil does not reduce total cholesterol levels as much as seed oils. In reality, it does very little to reduce harmful LDL cholesterol and total cholesterol. It does, however, raise HDL (beneficial cholesterol) levels.[34] This does not mean, however, that olive oil is less beneficial than seed oils, as was once thought. The use of olive oil provides *greater protection* against **arteriosclerosis** and **coronary disease** (angina and infarction) than *any other* oil, because it inhibits the oxidation of lipoproteins.

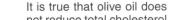
Olive oil

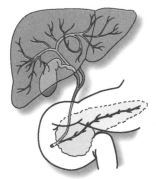

- **It inhibits the oxidation of lipoproteins.** It is known that the oxidation of low-density lipoproteins (a type of fat that circulates through the blood and contains a great deal of cholesterol), known by the initials LDL, is the *main* **mechanism** in the production of **arteriosclerosis**.

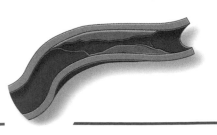

Numerous studies have demonstrated that *monounsaturated* fatty acids, such as oleic acid from olive oil, are more effective than *polyunsaturated* fatty acids in inhibiting oxidation of lipoproteins.[35, 36]

In other words, **olive oil** is *more effective* than those of **seeds** in the prevention of arteriosclerosis, even though seed oils reduce cholesterol levels to a greater degree.[37, 38, 39]

- **It reduces the risk of breast cancer.** Investigators from the Spanish National School of Health (Escuela Nacional de Sanidad, Madrid, Spain) were the first to propose that olive oil reduces the risk of breast cancer.[40] Another joint study by the University of Athens (Greece) and Harvard University (USA),[41] confirmed that an increase in olive oil consumption (more than once a day) lowered risk of breast cancer by 25% to 35%. On the other hand, the use of **margarine** is associated with a *higher* **risk** of this disease.

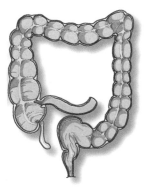

- **It protects the liver.** Olive oil promotes liver function and is *particularly* useful in case of some types of **hepatic insufficiency** due to hepatitis, cirrhosis or toxins from medications or from other sources. This has been confirmed experimentally with laboratory animals.[42]

It is equally useful in cases of **gallbladder** disorder due to its cholagogue effect (it aids drainage of the bile).

- **It helps avoid constipation.** It serves as *a mild, effective* laxative, particularly when it is taken on an empty stomach (one to two tablespoons are sufficient).

The Bitter Side of Sugar

Can it produce disease?

More Sugar and Less Fiber = Disease

Although sugar alone has no toxic or carcinogenic effects, there are studies that relate consumption of large amounts (more than 50 g a day) of sugar with various chronic diseases. It is possible that in many cases, the harmful effect of sugar is primarily due to a lack of fiber and certain vitamins and minerals displaced in the diet when a great deal of sugar and sugared products are eaten.[51]

This chart illustrates some of the diseases related to a diet that is high in sugar and low in fiber and other nutrients.

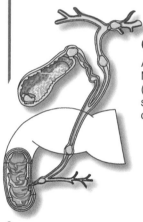

Gallstones

A long-term follow-up study conducted by the National Institute of Public Health in Bilthoven (Netherlands) showed a relationship between sugar consumption and increased risk of cholelithiasis.[50]

Crohn's Disease

The combination of a great deal of sugar and little fiber is one of the causative factors of this disease.[49]

Gastroduodenal Ulcer

The use of sugar, together with a diet of refined foods poor in fiber, increases this risk.[47]

Diabetes

There are no studies that prove that the liberal use of sugar is a cause of diabetes, but evidently it does make it worse and more serious.

Stomach Cancer

A study carried out in Marseilles (France) demonstrated that sugar, saturated fat, and, and, calcium increased the risk of stomach cancer. On the other hand, a diet that is rich in raw vegetables, fresh fruit, and vegetable oil reduces this risk.[48]

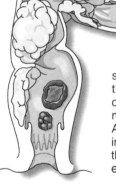

Colon Cancer

According to the Mario Negri Institute of Pharmacological Investigation in Milan (Italy), the consumption of sugar between meals stimulates the proliferation of the epithelial cells of the intestine.[43] This promotes the formation of cancers. Additionally, a study in Iowa (USA) involving 35,215 women found that the more sugar one eats the higher the risk of colon cancer.[44]

Bone Brittleness

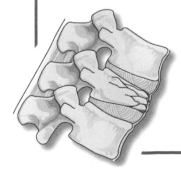

A high fat, high sugar diet depletes the calcium reserves in the body. This causes the bones to become brittle and fracture according to a study conducted at University of Southern California in Los Angeles (USA).[46]

Retarded Fetal Growth

A study at the University of New Jersey (USA) shows that pregnant adolescents who consume excess sugar, have a probability of giving birth to low weight babies.[45]

The Best Sweets: Fruit

Fruit is the most healthful way to eat sugars and satisfy the natural craving for sweets.

In Addition to Sugars, Fruits Contain:

- *Vitamins and minerals* that *facilitate* the **metabolism of sugar**, transforming it into energy.
- *Fiber,* which slows the absorption of sugars. For this reason, *less* **insulin** is required when eating fruit than when eating sugar alone or in refined products lacking fiber.

The less insulin is secreted, the *less* **fat** is produced, since one of insulin's effects is promotion of lipogenisis, in other words, the synthesis of lipids or fats in the body.

Due to all of this, the **natural** or intrinsic **sugar** found in fruit has two great advantages over extrinsic sugar added to foods, particularly if they are refined:

- it is better tolerated by diabetics,
- it is less fattening.

Calorie for calorie, natural fruit sugar is better utilized by the body and is less fattening than common sugar.

One large apple (200 g) = 25 g of sugar

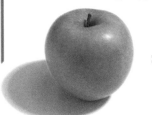 =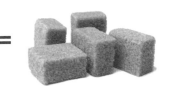

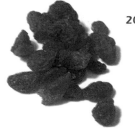 =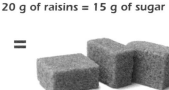
20 g of raisins = 15 g of sugar

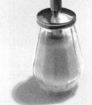 =
One dried fig (20 g) = 10 g of sugar

Nutritional Value of Different Natural Sweets

Very High
- **Dried fruits,** which **are** very rich in fiber, minerals, and vitamins.

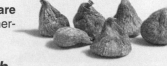

High
- **Molasses,** which is very rich in minerals, particularly iron and calcium.

Acceptable
- **Maple syrup, maple sugar, and brown sugar:** Contain small quantities of vitamins and minerals.

- **Honey,** in addition to being sweet, contains enzymes and proteins endowed with medicinal properties.

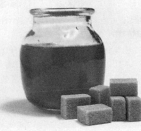

Low
- **Common sugar and other sugars** are almost completely void of nutritional elements. Thus its value is reduced to the *'empty'* **calories** that they contain.

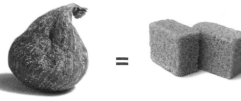

Alternatives

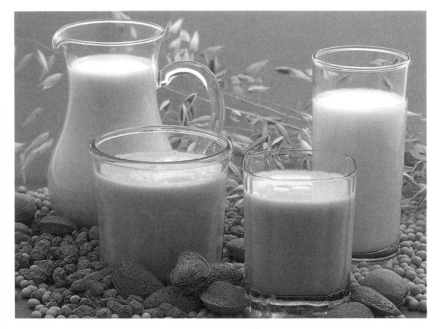

Alternatives to Cow's Milk

The so-called **'vegetable milks'** constitute *healthy and healthful* alternatives to milk.

- **Soy 'milk' or beverage:** This beverage does not naturally contain **vitamin B₁₂,** and has *less calcium* than cow's milk. However, **enriched** soy beverages are available whose nutritional value is very similar to cow's milk.

- **Almond 'milk' or beverage:** This very pleasant and refreshing beverage provides *proteins, unsaturated fats, and sugars* that are very easy to assimilate. It contains less *calcium* than cow's milk.

- **Oat 'milk' or beverage:** This is very rich in fats and proteins.

- **Tiger nut horchata:** Horchata contains *less protein* and calcium than milk, but more *carbohydrates, iron, and magnesium.*

Alternatives to Butter

- **Margarine:** Margarine as a substitute for butter has the *advantage* of containing **less saturated fat,** and *no cholesterol.* However, it has the disadvantage of containing a great deal of **'trans' fatty acids,** which promote arteriosclerosis.

- The healthiest **dietary** fat is neither butter nor margarine, but rather **cold-pressed olive oil** or **seed oils**.

Calcium Equivalents

Even though milk and dairy products are good sources of calcium, they **are not essential** in meeting the daily needs for this mineral.

One glass of milk (200 ml) = 100 g of almonds = 100 g of common dry beans = 500 g of broccoli

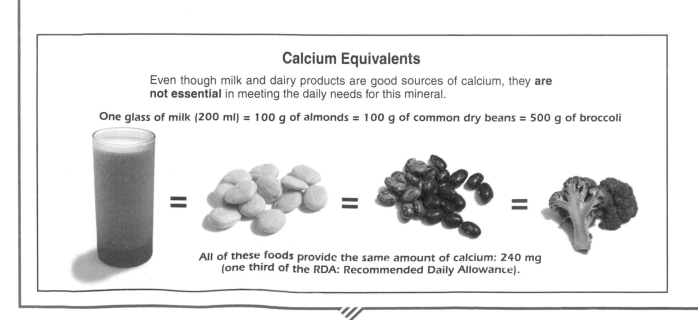

All of these foods provide the same amount of calcium: 240 mg
(one third of the RDA: Recommended Daily Allowance).

to Dairy Products

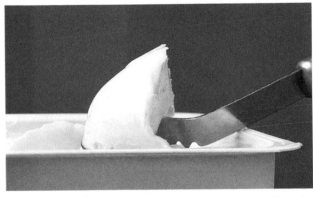

Margarine

Alternatives to Cheese

- **Tofu**: Tofu is made by coagulating soymilk. Its appearance, texture and nutritional value are similar to that of fresh cheeses. It contains 8% ***protein,*** and 105 mg/100 g of ***calcium;*** in other words, considerably more than **fresh cheeses** or **cottage cheese,** which contain between 65 and 70 mg/100 g of calcium.

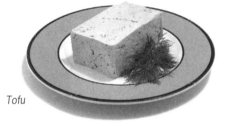

Tofu

Benefits of Alternatives to Dairy Products

- *They produce virtually **no** intolerance or **allergies.***
- *They do **not** present as high a **risk** of bacterial pathogenic **contamination** as milk, not do they contain **antibiotics** or **hormones.***
- *Their **fat** is predominantly **mono or polyunsaturated,** which contributes to the reduction of cholesterol and avoiding arteriosclerosis.*
- *They contain **no cholesterol.***
- *They contain **no lactose,** the milk sugar that causes intolerance.*

Reasons for Avoiding Dairy Products

There are more and more people who, for a variety of reasons that are generally

- **health**-related, or
- based on **ethical** considerations (respect for milk-producing animals, often over-exploited),

prefer not to consume milk and dairy products.

The food industry currently offers a variety of **vegetable products** that *can **replace** milk* and dairy products, although with lowered amounts of calcium and vitamin B$_{12}$, but with ***various and interesting** advantages,* as illustrated in these pages.

Milk Beverages

This is an alternative to regular milk that is made by:

- ***Eliminating** all of the milk **fat** and **cholesterol** from milk.*
- ***Adding** a **vegetable oil** (usually corn or soy), which is emulsified with the nonfat milk from the previous step.*
- ***Enriching** with liposoluble **vitamins A** and **D.***

Benefits

- *It retains the **nutritional value** and **flavor** of **whole milk.***
- *It is **rich in** vegetable unsaturated fatty acids. Contrary to the effect of milk's saturated fats, this actually **reduces the cholesterol level.***
- *It contains no cholesterol.*
- *It is **appropriate** for **patients with heart disease** and those who want to lower their **cholesterol** level: however, it is **not as effective** as **soy or almond milk.***

Eggs and Cholesterol

The egg has gotten a negative reputation due to its elevated cholesterol content. Is the egg as harmful to cardiovascular patients as had been thought?

The egg is the *richest* of animal products in **cholesterol** (425 mg/100 g). Only brain tissue is higher (2,200 mg/100 g).

The egg contains so much cholesterol because this lipid is indispensable for the development of the nervous system and endocrine glands of the embryo. However, **humans *do not* need** to take in cholesterol through their food, since the **liver** is capable of producing even more than the body needs.

One egg contains about 250 mg of cholesterol, an amount close to the 300 mg daily upper limit. This means that eating **one egg a day** and **any other animal product** (milk, meat, fish, etc.) substantially **surpasses** the 300 mg of cholesterol considered the maximum daily allowance.

Eggs Raise Cholesterol Only Slightly...

A study at the Copenhagen Clinic for the Study of Preventive Health (Denmark) demonstrates that eating two hard-boiled eggs a day for six weeks produces:[52]

* an *increase* in **HDL** cholesterol (beneficial) of 10%.
* a *slight increase* in **total** cholesterol of 4%.

If this is the case with two eggs a day, it is reasonable to say that **moderate consumption** of two or three eggs a week ***does not* raise** blood **cholesterol** level.

This and other discoveries confirm that the moderate use of eggs does not increase blood cholesterol level. In fact, cholesterol from food has a relatively limited impact on the blood levels of this lipid. **Saturated fat** *increases* cholesterol levels *more* than food cholesterol itself.

...But Promote Arteriosclerosis

Even though eggs do not raise blood cholesterol levels as much as was once thought, they do *promote* arteriosclerosis *to a greater degree* than was thought.

Cholesterol is only dangerous when it is deposited on the walls of arteries, which become hardened and narrower. Recent investigations have shown that this process, known as arteriosclerosis, is initiated by the oxidation of low-density lipoproteins (LDL), the substances transporting cholesterol in the blood plasma.

Studies conducted at the Rambam Medical Center in Haifa (Israel),[53] have shown that the consumption of two eggs a day for three weeks increases **oxidation of plasma lipoproteins** by 42%. This means that eggs promote the process of arterial deterioration and arteriosclerosis.

In addition to an increase in **cholesterol** level, other factors such as **smoking, lack of physical exercise,** or **obesity**, *contribute*, as well, to **lipoprotein oxidation** and to arteriosclerosis. *To the contrary*, **vegetables and fruit** rich in antioxidants *inhibit* this degenerative process.

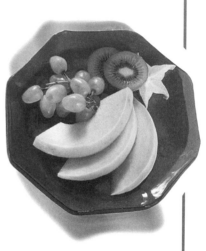

Prevention of Arteriosclerosis and Cardiovascular Disease

*Those at **high risk** for arteriosclerosis and cardiovascular disease in general because of high cholesterol levels or other causes, should:*

* **Avoid** eating **eggs**, and use **substitutes** in their place.
* **Discard the yolk** of the egg. The egg white contains no fats, and as has been shown,[136] its use reduces cholesterol levels.
* Use **eggs enriched** with omega-3 fatty acids, which do not increase cholesterol and reduce triglyceride levels.[137]
* **Never eat more than two eggs a week.**
* **Avoid fried eggs**, which supply more fat since they retain frying oil, thus promoting an increase in cholesterol.

The Egg and Hygiene

The egg is the ideal medium for the development of microorganisms. Although eggs contain protective membranes and antibacterial proteins such as lysozyme, many commercially available eggs are contaminated, even in developed countries.

A study conducted at the Institute of Social Medicine and Epidemiology in Berlin (Germany) shows that *Salmonella* bacteria in eggs are responsible for 67% of all food-related poisonings.[54]

Avoiding Egg-Transmitted Infections

- **Avoid eating raw eggs:** Sauces, particularly mayonnaise, are excellent media for the development of microorganisms from:
  - the egg itself
  - external contamination from hands, hair, and saliva of those handling the material during preparation.

  Pasteurized egg products should be used in place of raw eggs.[55]

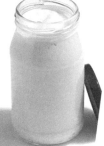

- **Discard eggs with cracked shells.** Intact eggs may be contaminated with salmonella[56] because bacteria penetrate the shell through its numerous pores. Those with damaged shells present an even greater risk of contamination.

- **Discard eggs contaminated with feces on the shell.** Washing does not eliminate the possibility of contamination, since the microbes have usually already entered the egg.

- **Store eggs in the refrigerator** and never longer than *three weeks.*

- **Use the freshest (most recently laid) eggs possible.** The longer an egg is stored, the greater the possibility that bacteria have developed in its interior.

How To Tell if an Egg Is Fresh

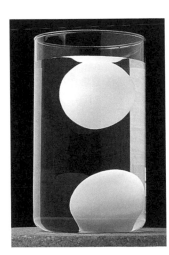

Recently laid eggs sink in water. As time passes, part of the water within the egg evaporates through the pores in the shell. This enlarges the air space in the egg and causes it to float.

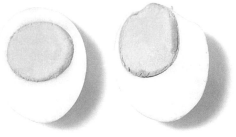

The yolk in recently laid eggs is found in the center. As the egg ages, the yolk moves to the side.

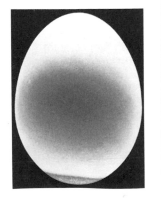

By observing a back-lit egg, one can see the size of the air space and the position of the yolk. As the egg ages, the separation between the yolk and the egg white becomes less distinct.

Potentially Toxic Portions of Fish

Blood: A **severe irritation** results from touching the **mouth** or **eyes** with hands contaminated with **eel, conger eel,** or **moray** blood. This often occurs while they are being cleaned.

Fins: Some species have spines in their dorsal fin that **inject poison** when touched.

Swim Bladder: This in itself is not toxic. However, it promotes bacterial contamination in fish. As it swells during the net-fishing process, it **compresses** the **stomach** and **intestine,** expelling their contaminated contents.

Skin: When it does *not* have **scales** and is **smooth,** it may contain **irritants;** in this case it *should be* handled with caution and **discarded** (lampreys, for example).

Liver: Fish liver contains *large amounts* of **vitamin A** in the form of retinol, which can cause **hypervitaminosis,** as opposed to provitamin A from plants.

Shark and **ray** livers are *particularly* toxic.

Stomach and Intestines: These organs harbor the larvae of the **anisakis** parasite, which perforates the walls of the digestive tract and enters the fish's flesh causing parasitosis and serious allergic reactions.

Roe: These are the **ovaries** of female fish at the time of egg-laying. They are *rich* in **fat** and *vitamins B$_1$ and B$_2$.*

About **40 species** of fish have been found to have **poisonous roe** without affecting the rest of the fish. These are primarily anadromous species (those that have marine and fluvial cycles), such as the **mullet** and the **salmon.**

Roe **poisoning** presents the following **symptoms:**

- **Digestive:** nausea, vomiting, diarrhea, dryness of the mouth;
- **General:** headache, fever, sweating, dizziness.

These symptoms tend to disappear after a few days. There is no specific treatment.

The **fish eggs** themselves are *not* toxic.

Fish and the Heart

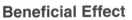

Beneficial Effect

Several epidemiological studies show that **regular consumption** of fish, whether lean or fatty, reduces the **risk** of heart attack (*myocardial infarction*). For example:

- A 30-year longitudinal study of 1,822 men in the United States demonstrated that those who ate a kilo of fish per month (one or two servings per week) showed 40% less risk of unexpected death due to heart attack (myocardial infarction).[57]
- Those who habitually eat fish or take fish-oil supplements suffer less arrhythmia and have a lower risk of sudden death due to cardiac arrest, particularly if they have had a previous heart attack (myocardial infarction).[58]

However, not only fish provides this effect. A diet rich in **linolenic acid** from vegetable sources (walnuts, flax-seed or soy products) produces the *same* results.[59]

Neutral or Negative Effect

These studies not withstanding, others find no benefit to fish. For example, a four-year longitudinal study of 44,895 North American male healthcare professionals shows that fish consumption or fish oil supplements have no bearing on heart attack risk.[60]

A study conducted in Finland, a country where fish consumption is traditionally high, provided some unexpected results: the more omega-3 fatty acids from fish sources, the greater the risk of death from heart disease such as myocardial infarction.[61]

In Summary

How can the apparent contradiction among these studies be explained?

Various facts help explain the effect of fish on the heart:

- If there is no corresponding *reduction* in the consumption of **saturated fats,** fish or fish oil will not protect against cardiovascular disease.[62]
- The **beneficial effects** of fish only become apparent **when it replaces** other foods in the diet which are high in saturated fats, such as meat. The idea is not so much to add fish to the diet, but to have fish **replace meat,** whose consumption is clearly harmful to the heart.

- The fact that heart attack risk is lowered regardless of whether lean or fatty fish are eaten leads to a conclusion that the beneficial effects are not due so much to fish oil (lean fish has very little), but rather to the fact that fish replaces other foods harmful to the heart.
- Fish, however, can be **harmful** to the cardiovascular system when:
  - it is **contaminated** with high levels of **mercury,**
  - it is **contaminated** with **bacteria** that produce histamine and other vasoactive biogenic amines.
  - It contains a *great* deal of **salt,** as is the case with certain preserving techniques.

Better Than Fish

- **Fish** is **beneficial** to the **heart** if it is accompanied by a *reduction* in **meat.**
- Fish is *not necessary* for a healthy heart.

  Vegetable foods such as fruit, whole grains, and legumes provide *more protective* substances to the **heart** than fish, but with *fewer* drawbacks.

Meat-related Cancers

*Recent studies associate regular meat consumption
with these types of cancer:*

Cancer of the Mouth and Pharynx

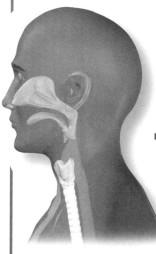

Although the *most important* risk factors for these cancers are **smoking** and **drinking alcoholic beverages,** eating **salted** or **cured meat** also influences its genesis, according to studies conducted in Uruguay.[68]

Colon Cancer

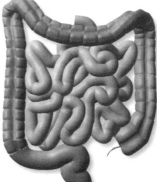

Men who eat red meat (beef, pork, or lamb) as a main dish five or more times a week have four times greater risk of colon cancer than those that eat these meats less than once a month. This is the result of a broad statistical study conducted at the School of Public Health at Harvard University (Massachusetts, USA).[64]

Eating 600 grams (1.32 pounds) of red meat—but not white meat (chicken) or fish—triples the amount of N-nitrous compounds in the feces, which explains the **carcinogenic *effect*** of **red meat** on the colon, according to the Medical Research Council of Cambridge (UK).[65]

A *high* intake of animal **fat** also increases the risk of colon cancer.[66]

Kidney Cancer

Carcinoma in renal cells is more frequent with greater fat, meat, and meat products, according to the German Institute of Human Nutrition in Bergholz-Rehbrucke.[63]

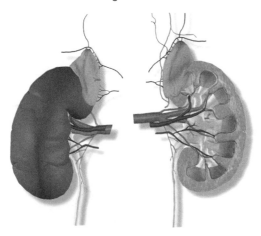

Breast Cancer

Women who eat meat more than five times a week run a two and a half times greater risk of breast cancer than those who eat it two times a week or less, according to the Montebello Institute of Epidemiological Investigation (Oslo, Norway).[67]

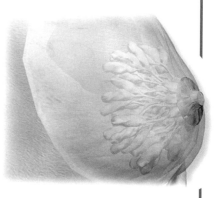

Is Meat Addictive?

The stimulant hypoxanthine, not any special properties of its protein, vitamins, or minerals, is responsible for the satisfying and stimulating effects of meat. It is similar in chemical formula and effect to caffeine.

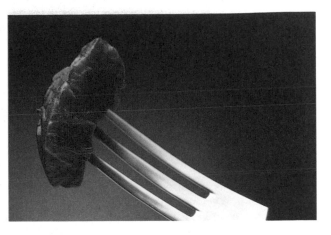

It has been known since antiquity that those who regularly eat meat experience some degree of enervation when they are deprived of this food for some time.

This sensation that "something is missing" always results from abruptly removing meat from the diet, even when it is replaced with plant foods and dietary supplements providing as much or even more protein and nutrients as meat.

A Stimulant in Meat

The enervation that some persons experience when they stop eating meat products is not due to lack of its protein or other nutrients that some consider irreplaceable. It is due to a type of stimulant found in meat.

Today it is known that the muscle cells of meat contain **hypoxanthine,** which increases in concentration as the meat ages. Hypoxanthine is formed by:

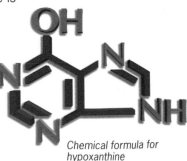

Chemical formula for hypoxanthine

- The degradation of ATP (adenosine triphosphate),
- The decomposition of the nucleotides that form DNA and RNA in the nuclei of the cells.

The Effects of Hypoxanthine

Hypoxanthine and other similar substances, such as **inosinic acid** and **guanylic acid,** are present in meat. They have a chemical structure *similar* to that of **caffeine** in coffee or the **theobromine** in cocoa, with similar effects. For example:

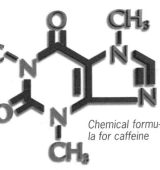

Chemical formula for caffeine

- They are **central nervous system stimulants** that produce a sensation of vitality and energy, which in many cases is simply a feeling.

- They **are addictive,** meaning that use must be continued in order to avoid withdrawal symptoms.

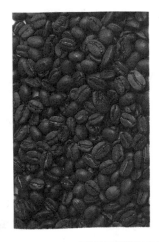

Hypoxanthine explains the stimulating effect of meat and its capacity to create a certain level of addiction, which manifests itself when meat is given up abruptly. Because of this, it is recommended that those wishing to replace meat with plant-based foods follow a transition diet to help avoid the effects of sudden deprivation.

Meat is not essential in the human diet. By understanding the nutritional value of the available alternatives, eliminating it can be easy and healthful.

Legumes

A plate of legumes can substitute for a serving of meat in terms of nutrition:

- **Protein:** Legumes provide protein that is **equal to or superior** to that of meat in *quality* and *quantity*. However, the digestibility of legume protein is not as good as that of meat. The **biological value** of meat protein as well as that of legumes is *increased* when it is **combined** with that of **grains** (supplementation).

- **Iron:** Legumes generally provide *more* **iron** than meat. This availability compensates for the fact that the iron from legumes is less absorbable.

- **Other differences:** Legumes are a good source of **carbohydrates** and **fiber,** which are missing in meat. Additionally, they do **not** contain **cholesterol.** On the other hand, legumes lack **vitamin B₁₂,** which is abundant in meat.

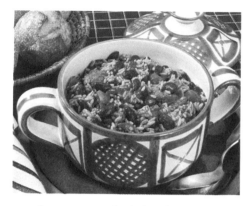

Legumes, particularly when combined with grains, are comparable or even superior to meat in terms of protein and minerals; although not in vitamin B₁₂.

Vegetable "Meat"

This is a healthy and delicious alternative to meat. It may be prepared at home from a variety of ingredients such as **soy, oatmeal, nuts, or gluten.** Methods of preparation are explained in detail in the accompanying book of recipes.

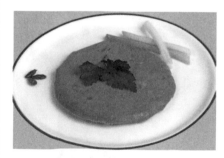

Soy Protein

Texturized soy protein has a texture similar to that of meat. It is essentially flavorless, which necessitates its preparation with other vegetables to make "hamburgers," "meat" balls, fillings and other dishes similar to those made with meat.

Their **nutritional value** and **flavor** can be *equal* to or *superior* to those of **meat.**

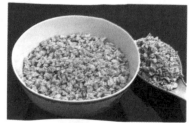

Oil-bearing Nuts

These constitute an alternative to meat because they are rich in **protein, minerals,** and **vitamins**.

Gluten

Gluten is **protein** extracted from **wheat** or other **grains** . It is used in a variety of meatless recipes. Its flavor is neutral so it must be prepared and flavored. Gluten has two important *drawbacks:*

- There are persons who suffer from **celiac disease** (gluten intolerance).

- It is an **incomplete** **protein** and must be complemented by other vegetable proteins.

Soy Derivatives

Tofu, tempeh (contains vitamin B₁₂) and *miso* present many **advantages** as meat analogs.

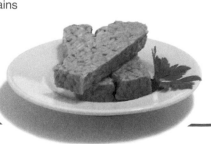

Alternatives

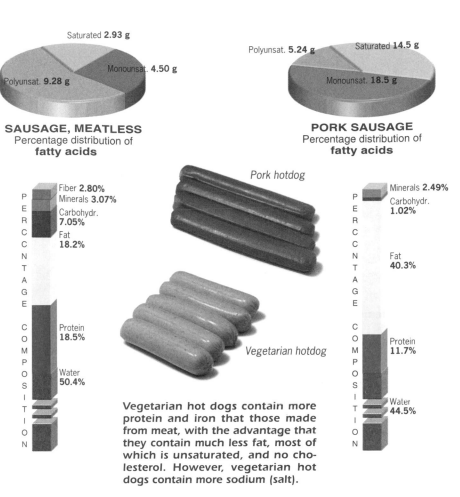

SAUSAGE, MEATLESS
Percentage distribution of **fatty acids**

Saturated **2.93 g**
Monounsat. **4.50 g**
Polyunsat. **9.28 g**

PORK SAUSAGE
Percentage distribution of **fatty acids**

Polyunsat. **5.24 g**
Saturated **14.5 g**
Monounsat. **18.5 g**

P E R C E N T A G E   C O M P O S I T I O N

Fiber **2.80%**
Minerals **3.07%**
Carbohydr. **7.05%**
Fat **18.2%**
Protein **18.5%**
Water **50.4%**

Minerals **2.49%**
Carbohydr. **1.02%**
Fat **40.3%**
Protein **11.7%**
Water **44.5%**

Pork hotdog

Vegetarian hotdog

Meat Analogs

Meat analogs are prepared from a soy base. They are useful for those seeking a **transitional diet** from meat to one based on plant foods.

For those whose diet is already formed around vegetables, they can be an occasional complement, but they *should not* constitute *a dietary base.*

Benefits

All of those associated with plant-based foods as opposed to animal-based foods.

- *No* **cholesterol;**
- They contain *mostly* **unsaturated** *fats;*
- They provide *carbohydrates* and in some cases, vegetable *fiber;*
- They do not have the **carcinogenic effect** of meat.

Drawbacks:

- They are **processed foods,** which are generally made from **refined products.** They contain added **salt** and, in *some cases,* **additives** (thickeners, preservatives, and antioxidants). It is important to note, however, that many of these additives are of natural origin.

- *They can be* **difficult to digest,** since they are *concentrated* foods and contain **spices** to compensate for the neutral flavor of the soy protein.

Vegetarian hot dogs contain more protein and iron that those made from meat, with the advantage that they contain much less fat, most of which is unsaturated, and no cholesterol. However, vegetarian hot dogs contain more sodium (salt).

SAUSAGE, MEATLESS
Composition
per 100 g of raw edible portion

Energy	256 kcal = 1072 kj
Protein	18.5 g
Carbohydrates	7.05 g
Fiber	2.80 g
Vitamin A	64.0 µg RE
Vitamin B₁	2.34 mg
Vitamin B₂	0.402 mg
Niacin	15.8 mg NE
Vitamin B₆	0.828 mg
Folate	26.0 µg
Vitamin B₁₂	—
Vitamin C	—
Vitamin E	2.10 mg α-TE
Calcium	63.0 mg
Phosphorus	225 mg
Magnesium	36.0 mg
Iron	3.72 mg
Potassium	231 mg
Zinc	1.46 mg
Total Fat	18.2 g
Saturated Fat	2.93 g
Cholesterol	—
Sodium	888 mg

1%   2%   4%   10%   20%   40%   100%
% Daily Value (based on a 2,000 calorie diet)
provided by 100 g of this food

PORK SAUSAGE
Composition
per 100 g of raw edible portion

Energy	417 kcal = 1746 kj
Protein	11.7 g
Carbohydrates	1.02 g
Fiber	—
Vitamin A	—
Vitamin B₁	0.545 mg
Vitamin B₂	0.164 mg
Niacin	4.40 mg NE
Vitamin B₆	0.250 mg
Folate	4.00 µg
Vitamin B₁₂	1.13 µg
Vitamin C	2.00 mg
Vitamin E	—
Calcium	18.0 mg
Phosphorus	118 mg
Magnesium	11.0 mg
Iron	0.910 mg
Potassium	204 mg
Zinc	1.59 mg
Total Fat	40.3 g
Saturated Fat	14.5 g
Cholesterol	68.0 mg
Sodium	667 mg

1%   2%   4%   10%   20%   40%   100%
% Daily Value (based on a 2,000 calorie diet)
provided by 100 g of this food

Types of Salt

Sea Salt

In *addition* to **sodium chloride**, sea salt contains *small amounts* of the salts of **calcium, potassium,** and **magnesium**. These are very beneficial minerals that partially compensate for the harmful effects of excess sodium. Sea salt also provides a *small* but **important** amount of **iodine**.

The **drawback** to unrefined sea salt is that it *retains* a lot of **moisture,** which makes it harder to handle. But its benefits far outweigh this small inconvenience.

Refined Salt

This is *more* **common** but *less* **healthful**. It is prepared by:

• **Removing** the **magnesium** and **calcium** salts that sea salt naturally contains and that cause the salt to clump. This makes the salt easier to use both for the packager and in the kitchen, but at the cost of the mineral content of sea salt.

• Various **additives** are *used* to keep the salt grains free and dry.

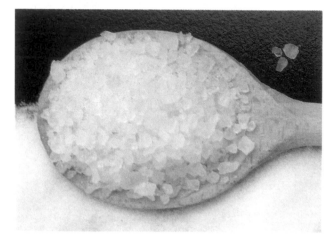

A few grains of rice mixed with salt absorb the moisture it may contain making it easier to pour.

The Need For Salt

The average Western diet provides **eight times** more salt and sodium than the body **needs.**

For some persons, salt can become a "**drug**" almost as dangerous as alcohol or tobacco. Aside from its harmful health effects, salt has the ability to become habit-forming.

Approximately half a teaspoon of salt a day, 1.25 g, covers the need for sodium of an adult with a sedentary lifestyle. The foods that normally make up the diet provide more than enough sodium without a need to add salt.

Those involved in intense physical labor or who live in hot climates need more salt: approximately one gram per each hour of sweating.

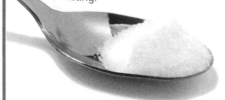

	Sodium (mg)	Equivalent in common salt (g)*
Minimum daily needs of an adult	500	1.25
Daily Value (acceptable daily intake)	2,400	6
Normal consumption	4,000	10

* Equivalents:
  1 g of salt contains 0.4 g of sodium (400 mg).
  1 g of sodium (1,000 mg) equals 2.5 g of salt.

Than a Seasoning

"Hidden Salt": An Abundant Additive

Grams of salt contained in 100 grams of each of these products:

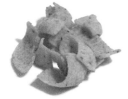

Fast food and snacks: 2-3 g

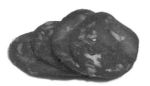

Sausages and cured meats: 3-6 g

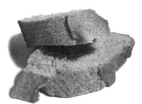

Bread:[71] 1.2 g

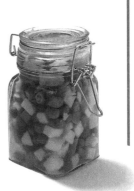

Preserves: 1-2 g

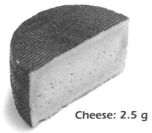

Cheese: 2.5 g

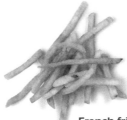

French-fried potatoes: 2.5 g

Bottled tomato juice: 1.125 g

Just as with sugar it is possible that the *worst* aspect of salt may not be the sodium chloride itself but the *unhealthful* foods usually **accompanying** it: cured meats, sausages, fried foods, refined products (without fiber), etcetera. These foods *trigger* the **harmful effects** of salt.

There are many specialists, such as Professor Mac-Gregor of the Hypertension Unit of Saint George Hospital in London, who see a clear connection between excess use of common salt (NaCl, sodium chloride) and arterial hypertension, strokes, and osteoporosis. They all question why the food industry is so loath to reduce the amount of salt added to precooked dishes, preserves and other processed foods.[69, 70]

Salt Alternatives

To reduce the use of salt, one must **first accustom the palate** to a less intense salt taste. The following alternatives may be useful:

- **Other salts such as potassium chloride and potassium iodide.** These have a somewhat less salty taste than sodium chloride. They are usually mixed with it to form dietetic salts. **Diabetics** and those suffering from **renal failure** must use them with care since an excess of **potassium** may be harmful in these cases.

- **Herb salt** contains a mixture of common salt, **other salts** and **aromatic herb extracts**. It contains approximately **half** the **sodium** of the common salt by weight. Its flavor is somewhat less salty than common salt, but it is tastier due to the aromatic herbs.

- **Healthful seasonings** provide flavor and health (lemon, aromatic herbs, garlic, onion, etc.).

- **Sea salt,** although it contains practically the same amount of **sodium** as refined salt, it is somewhat less **harmful** because it contains other **minerals** that partially **compensate** for the undesirable effects of sodium.

Fruit-flavored Beverages

Almost all are **carbonated** and are referred to as **sodas**. They *lack nutritional value* except the sugar they contain (90-120 g/l).

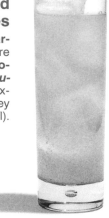

Tonic Water

These are sweetened (80-100 grams of sugar per liter, about 1.5 ounces per pint) carbonated beverages, which contain fruit **extracts** and a small amount of **quinine** (45-85 mg/l). Quinine is an alkaloid extracted from the quinine tree endowed with fever reducing, antimalarial, and invigorating effects.[72]

Tonic water contains no caffeine or phosphoric acid.

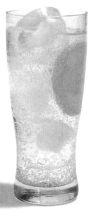

Cola Beverages

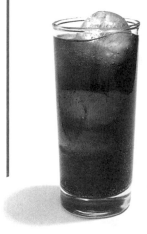

These contain **sugar** or chemical **sweeteners, carbon dioxide**, a variety of natural **extracts, phosphoric acid**, and **caffeine**. They are simply unhealthful with *many **drawbacks.***

Cola beverages are *particularly **undesirable*** for **children** and for those suffering from **insomnia** or **cardiac disease** because of their caffeine content.

The Calories in a Can of Soft Drink

A ***330 ml*** *(11 ounces) can of soft drink, either cola or fruit-flavored, sweetened with sugar contains around* ***35 g*** *(1.25 ounces)* ***of sugar***, *which provides* ***140 calories***, *approximately the same as:*

- ***55 g*** *(2 ounces) of* ***bread,***
- ***400 ml*** *(about 1 pint) of* ***nonfat milk,*** *or*
- ***240 g*** *(about half a pound) of* ***apples*** *(two medium-sized apples).*

However, the calories in soft drinks have a serious drawback: they are ***"empty."*** *This means that vitamins or minerals do not accompany them. Because of this, they* ***foster obesity and upset metabolism.***

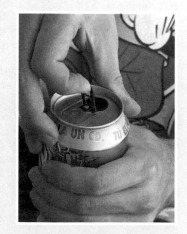

"Bitters"

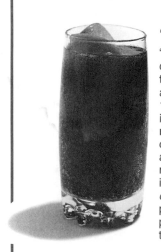

"Bitters" are *similar* in composition to **tonic water**, but with less quinine and more sugar (up to 135 g/l). Their characteristic ingredient is a **bitter natural extract**, which increases the **appetite and** aids **digestion**. Their primary drawback, however, is that *their high* **sugar** *content* **counteracts** *any* possible health benefits provided by the plant extracts.

Without Nutritional Value

Drawbacks to Soft Drinks

- **They are *not* thirst-quenching:** Because of sugar content and other chemical substances, many soft drinks leave an after-thirst. This leads to even greater thirst than before.

- **"Empty" calories:** Sugar-sweetened soft drinks contain many calories, which are **"empty"** (see box on previous page). In order for the **sugar** in a soft drink to be *transformed* into **energy**, *B-group vitamins* and *minerals* are *essential*. Since these are absent in soft drinks, they must be obtained from the body's own reserves, thus depleting them. In situations where the individual is not involved in physical exercise, this sugar is *turned to* **fat**.

- **Stomach irritation:** Some degree of irritation and inflammation of the mucous lining of the stomach is associated with the digestive process of carbonated beverages. Soft drinks *should be avoided* in cases of **gastritis**, gastroduodenal **ulcer**, and digestive **disorders** in general.

- **Dental caries:** The combination of sugar and acids such as phosphoric acid and others attack dental enamel *very* **aggressively**. Soft drink consumption is a causal factor in dental caries.[73]

- **Decalcification:** Several acids, including phosphoric acid, are added to cola beverages. Phosphoric acid **acidifies** the blood, which the body attempts to neutralize by releasing calcium and other minerals from the bones. That is why cola beverages have a decalcifying action and *should be particularly* **avoided** in cases of **rickets** and **osteoporosis**.

- **Allergies:** Many of the additives in soft drinks can cause allergies, which may manifest in many ways:
  – skin eruptions,
  – stomach pain and digestive disorders,
  – nervous irritability and hyperactivity.

- **Urinary stones:** *Regular* **consumption** of cola **beverages** *increases* the **risk** of urinary stones. This is because they foster elimination of calcium and oxalates through the urine. These substances form most urinary stones.[74]

Benefits of Soft Drinks

- **Water content:** From a health standpoint, the *only* **positive** aspect of soft drinks is their **water** content. By drinking soft drinks one is drinking water, which improves kidney function.

- **Stimulate digestion:** The carbonation in soft drinks *irritates* the stomach mucosa *to some degree*, resulting in *increased* **gastric juice** *production*, which speeds digestion.

- **They do *not* contain alcohol.**

The nutritional value of soft drinks is virtually nonexistent, except the sugar they contain. Their many additives present a health risk.

In reality, the only positive aspect to soft drinks is their water content.

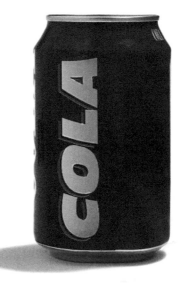

Coffee: a Stimulating

Coffee is a highly aromatic stimulant beverage prepared from roasted and ground coffee beans. Coffee beans are the seeds of the *Coffea arabica* or the *Coffea robusta* plants.

Coffee is a *true* **drug** due to its caffeine content. It meets the criteria set by the World Health Organization (WHO) for drug addiction:

- It creates **addiction** or dependency;
- Produces **tolerance** (the dose must be increased to achieve the same effect);
- Its elimination results in **abstinence syndrome**;
- Its *regular* **use** is **harmful** to health.

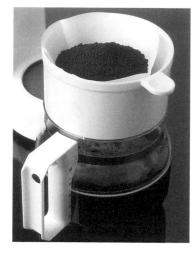

Coffee-drinking raises cholesterol levels. However, this effect is eliminated when it is brewed using a paper filter. The substance that raises cholesterol is not caffeine, but rather an aromatic substance in the coffee that remains in the paper filter.[75, 76]

Contents of a Cup of Coffee

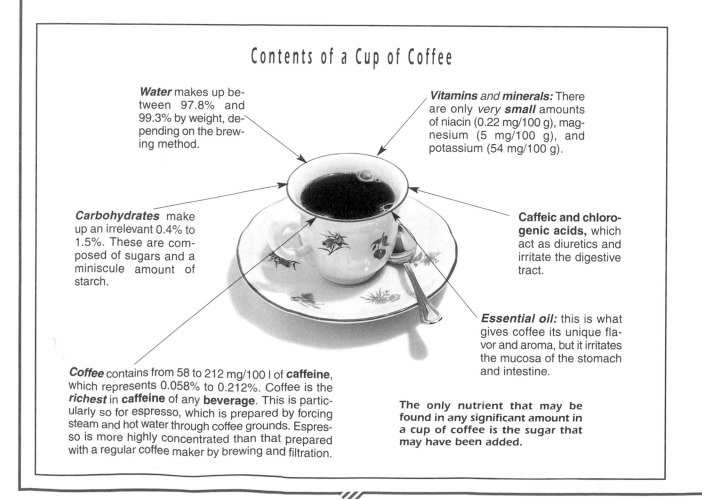

Water makes up between 97.8% and 99.3% by weight, depending on the brewing method.

Vitamins and **minerals:** There are only *very* **small** amounts of niacin (0.22 mg/100 g), magnesium (5 mg/100 g), and potassium (54 mg/100 g).

Carbohydrates make up an irrelevant 0.4% to 1.5%. These are composed of sugars and a miniscule amount of starch.

Caffeic and chlorogenic acids, which act as diuretics and irritate the digestive tract.

Essential oil: this is what gives coffee its unique flavor and aroma, but it irritates the mucosa of the stomach and intestine.

Coffee contains from 58 to 212 mg/100 l of **caffeine**, which represents 0.058% to 0.212%. Coffee is the **richest** in **caffeine** of any **beverage**. This is particularly so for espresso, which is prepared by forcing steam and hot water through coffee grounds. Espresso is more highly concentrated than that prepared with a regular coffee maker by brewing and filtration.

The only nutrient that may be found in any significant amount in a cup of coffee is the sugar that may have been added.

and Aromatic Drug

Harmful Effects of Coffee

The harmfulness of coffee is the subject of broad debate among researchers. While some feel that moderate amounts (2 to 3 cups a day) is safe, others are equally certain that it produces numerous disorders.

This page illustrates its proven harmful effects, which it has in common with other stimulant beverages.

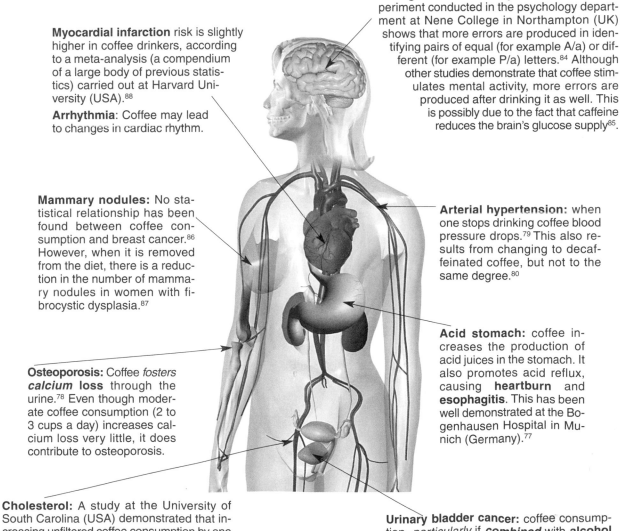

Myocardial infarction risk is slightly higher in coffee drinkers, according to a meta-analysis (a compendium of a large body of previous statistics) carried out at Harvard University (USA).[88]

Arrhythmia: Coffee may lead to changes in cardiac rhythm.

Changes in intellectual performance: An experiment conducted in the psychology department at Nene College in Northampton (UK) shows that more errors are produced in identifying pairs of equal (for example A/a) or different (for example P/a) letters.[84] Although other studies demonstrate that coffee stimulates mental activity, more errors are produced after drinking it as well. This is possibly due to the fact that caffeine reduces the brain's glucose supply[85].

Mammary nodules: No statistical relationship has been found between coffee consumption and breast cancer.[86] However, when it is removed from the diet, there is a reduction in the number of mammary nodules in women with fibrocystic dysplasia.[87]

Arterial hypertension: when one stops drinking coffee blood pressure drops.[79] This also results from changing to decaffeinated coffee, but not to the same degree.[80]

Acid stomach: coffee increases the production of acid juices in the stomach. It also promotes acid reflux, causing **heartburn** and **esophagitis**. This has been well demonstrated at the Bogenhausen Hospital in Munich (Germany).[77]

Osteoporosis: Coffee *fosters calcium loss* through the urine.[78] Even though moderate coffee consumption (2 to 3 cups a day) increases calcium loss very little, it does contribute to osteoporosis.

Cholesterol: A study at the University of South Carolina (USA) demonstrated that increasing unfiltered coffee consumption by one cup a day on a regular basis raises blood cholesterol by 20 mg/100 ml.[83]

Urinary bladder cancer: coffee consumption, *particularly* if **combined** with **alcohol** use, significantly raises the risk of this type of cancer.[81, 82]

What Is Not Said

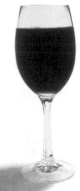

Scientific investigation has uncovered more negative aspects than positive to wine and other alcoholic beverages, even in low to moderate doses. However, these are seldom spoken of.

Various statistical studies have shown that drinking one or two small glasses of wine a day may reduce myocardial infarction risk in men fifty years old and older.

However, many other studies demonstrate that moderate consumption of wine or other alcoholic beverages increases risk of arterial hypertension, esophageal reflux, gastritis, liver disease, and various types of cancer, among other diseases.

So the benefit-risk ratio for wine is much lower than reported. Compared to unfermented grape juice, wine offers very little benefit at a very high risk.

 ## Positive Aspects of Wine

- **Stimulates digestion:** Alcohol *irritates* the mucosa of the digestive tract much in the same way it irritates the tissue of a wound on the skin. The cells of the stomach's mucosa secrete more juices to counteract this irritation. This, in turn, promotes digestion. In other words, the digestive stimulation produced by alcohol is at the expense of *irritation and inflammation* of the stomach mucosa, which can result in **gastritis**, gastroduodenal **ulcer**, or **cancer** of the esophagus or stomach. These diseases are more common among drinkers, even moderate drinkers.

- **Beneficial action on the heart:** Various statistical studies show that drinking between *100 and 200 ml* (1/2-1 cup) of red wine a day (not white wine) lowers the risk of death from heart attack.[89, 90, 91] This effect *only* seems to involve *men* over the *age of 50*.

These same statistics report that when more than this amount of wine (*200 ml* or about 1 cup of wine or 20 g of pure alcohol) is *exceeded,* the **mortality rate** due to **cardiovascular** disease *increases*, and *many other disorders* are fostered.[92]

The possible beneficial effect of red wine has been attributed to two of its ingredients:

– **Ethyl alcohol**: Some statistical studies have shown that any alcoholic beverage, even in small amounts, has a protective effect on the heart.[93] However, experiments conducted with laboratory animals show that only high blood alcohol levels, at least 2 grams per liter (2 g/l) of blood, is enough to reduce the platelets' tendency to clot within the arteries.[94] In other words, in order for alcohol to affect blood clotting positively, one would need to be intoxicated, with all of the health concerns that entails.

Smaller amounts of alcohol, such as one or two glasses of wine a day, have been proved insufficient to protect the cardiovascular system.

– *Phenolic flavonoids:* these substances come from the grape and its skin, which give red wine its color.[95] They act to inhibit the oxidation of lipoproteins, and by so doing, prevent cholesterol deposits within the arteries known as **arteriosclerosis**.[96] **Fruit** in general, and **grapes** in *particular*, are the *best* sources of *flavonoids*.

In other words, whatever small benefit may come from wine is from the grape. Eating **grapes** themselves or drinking **grape juice** is *much more **healthful*** for the heart and the entire body.

About Wine

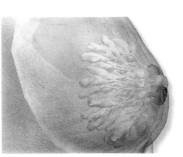

Women who drink alcoholic beverages, including wine, even in small amounts, are at higher risk for breast cancer and other disorders.

Drawbacks to Wine and Other Alcoholic Beverages

Virtually *everyone* **recognizes** that consuming **large amounts** of alcohol is **harmful**. However, numerous studies confirm undesirable effects of even reduced amounts of alcohol, such as the wine recommended to reduce heart attack risk:

- **Cerebral hemorrhage** is more frequent among drinkers.[97]
- **Arterial hypertension:** It has been shown that three or more glasses of wine a day can increase arterial pressure, which represents a risk factor to the cardiovascular system.[98]
- **Cancer in general** is more frequent among moderate drinkers than nondrinkers.[99]
- **Colon cancer** is also more frequent among those who drink moderately than those who do not drink at all.[100]
- **Breast cancer:** Women who consume moderate amounts of alcohol are at higher risk of breast cancer, as is confirmed by studies throughout the world. For example:
  - The University of Milan (Italy) has verified that women who drink 24.3 g of alcohol (one-fourth liter or 1 cup of wine, approximately) or more a day, are at twice the risk of breast cancer than nondrinkers.[101]
  - A study in the United States involving 89,539 women showed that those who consumed 15 g of alcohol a day (about 150 ml of wine) are at 2.5 times higher risk of breast cancer than those who do not drink.[102]
- **Stomach cancer:** The relationship between alcohol use and cancers of the esophagus and the stomach has been well known for many years. The General Direction of Health in Portugal conducted a study to quantify this relationship. It was observed that the greater the wine consumption, the higher the risk of stomach cancer:[103]
  - Drinkers that consume less than one glass of wine with a meal are at a 36% higher risk than nondrinkers.

  - Those who consume a bottle or more a day are at almost four times greater risk than nondrinkers.
- **Esophageal reflux:** The Clinic Hospital of Barcelona (Spain) has confirmed that men who drink 360 ml of wine during meals (somewhat less than two glasses) experience 70% more esophageal reflux than those who drink the same amount of water. Reflux is the ascension of the acid content of the stomach into the esophagus, causing heartburn (a burning sensation and inflammation of the esophagus, called esophagitis).[104]
- **Bone fracture:** women who drink 25 grams of alcohol (one large glass of wine) or more a day are at 2.33 times greater risk of hip fracture than those who do not drink.[105] Moderate amounts of alcohol, as well as coffee, promote osteoporosis and possible bone fractures.
- **Fetal alterations:** Pregnant women who drink 400 ml (two glasses) or more of wine a day, or its equivalent in other alcoholic beverages, have a higher incidence than nondrinkers of:[106]
  - Premature births,
  - Low birthweight babies, and
  - Immature placentas.

  Greater amounts of alcohol during pregnancy affect the fetus even more seriously and may lead to birth defects (fetal alcohol syndrome).
- **Other diseases:** Alcohol consumption is associated with *higher* **risk** of **cirrhosis** of the liver, **cerebral atrophy, arrhythmia, cardiomyopathy** (degeneration of the heart muscle itself), and **gout**.

Any **possible** *benefit* that *small* **amounts** of wine or other alcoholic beverage may have on the heart is far *outweighed* by its **drawbacks**. As a result, the World Health Organization and other specialists state categorically that alcohol intake as a prophylaxis for heart disease should not be promoted as a public health measure. In other words, *no* **health benefits** are obtained by **recommending** that *nondrinkers* should *drink* a little wine.[107, 108]

By substituting each of these foods with the one to its right, it is possible to reduce cholesterol levels. The more substitutions are made, the greater the cholesterol reduction. Additionally, following the counsels regarding arteriosclerosis will prove of benefit.

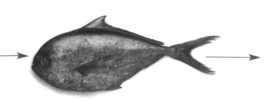
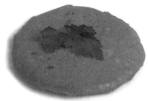

Red Meat, Shellfish, Sausages

Red meats are beef, lamb, and pork. They promote increases in cholesterol levels and arteriosclerosis.
Crustacean shellfish contain almost twice the cholesterol as meat in addition to having other drawbacks.

Fish or Skinless Poultry

These contain fats that are less prejudicial than those of red meat, although they cannot be said to reduce cholesterol. They are only beneficial when they **replace** *red meat or shellfish.*

Legumes, Meat Analogs, and Other Alternatives to Meat

These contain no cholesterol or fat that fosters its production in the body. Additionally, legumes contain soluble fiber that reduces cholesterol level and prevents arteriosclerosis.

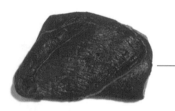
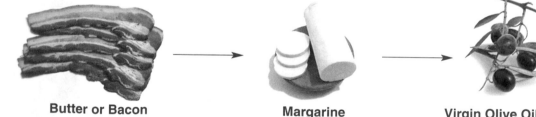
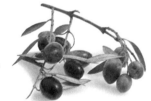

Butter or Bacon

Being very rich in saturated fat and cholesterol, these products are the most harmful for arterial health.

Margarine

When it **replaces** *butter, bacon or animal fat in general, margarine reduces cholesterol.[138] However, it contains trans fatty acids that foster arteriosclerosis.*

Virgin Olive Oil or Seed Oils

Both are more healthful than margarine and reduce cholesterol levels when they **replace** *margarine in the diet.[138]*
Olive oil *does not reduce cholesterol level as much as that of seeds (corn, soy, etc.), but it protects against arteriosclerosis, which, in the end, is more important.*

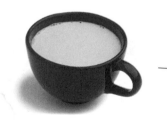
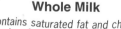
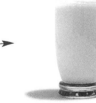
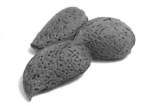

Whole Milk

This contains saturated fat and cholesterol. The casein of milk increases cholesterol levels as well.

Nonfat Milk

This is preferable to whole milk, but its casein content still has a negative effect on cholesterol level.

Soy or Almond Milk

These contain no cholesterol, lactose, or casein, all of which are detrimental to cardiovascular health. Soymilk also contains cardioprotective isoflavones (phytoestrogens).

Foods To
Cholesterol

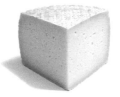

Cured Cheese

This contains **saturated fat, cholesterol** and **sodium,** all of which are prejudicial to arterial health.

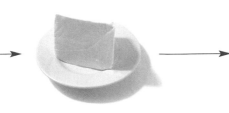

Low-fat Cottage Cheese

This is **preferable** to cured cheese, but not as healthful as tofu or avocado.

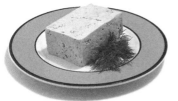

Tofu and Avocado

These are an excellent replacement for cheese. They **both** reduce cholesterol level. Avocado provides antioxidant vitamin E.

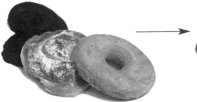

Industrial Pastries and Sweet Rolls

These contain refined **sugars** and **trans fatty acids,** which increase cholesterol and foster arteriosclerosis.

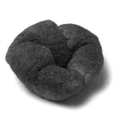

Whole-Grain Baked Goods

Preferably made without hydrogenated vegetable oils, thus eliminating trans fatty acids.

Sweets, Chocolate

The **sugar** and **fat** they contain increase cholesterol level.

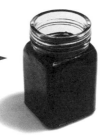

Dried Fruit, Honey, Molasses

These are the most healthful of sweets.

Types of Fatty Acids

- **Saturated fatty acids:** These are found in milk, egg yolk, and meat and its derivatives. They increase cholesterol production in the body.

  - **Medium chain saturated fatty acids:** These acids are found in some plant foods such as coconuts, and **do not** increase cholesterol production as do other saturated fatty acids.

- **Unsaturated fatty acids:**
  - *Monounsaturated* such as **oleic acid** found in olive oil: They **reduce LDL** (harmful) cholesterol and increase **HDL,** which *protects* against **arteriosclerosis.**

  - *Polyunsaturated:* These are found primarily in seed oils. They reduce LDL (harmful) cholesterol. **Omega-3** fatty acids are a special type of polyunsaturated fatty acid present specifically in fatty fish.

- **Trans fatty acids:** These are unsaturated fatty acids **altered** by **heat** or industrial processes. They are formed when **frying** with vegetable oils or when they are processed industrially by heating and **hydrogenation** to produce **semisolid fats** such as **margarine.**

  - Products that **contain them: hydrogenated vegetable oils, margarine, sauces, industrial baked goods,** and **fried foods.** The food industry prefers these because they **do not become rancid** as easily as vegetable oil.

  - **Health effects:** Trans fatty acids *increase* **LDL** (harmful) **cholesterol,** *reduce* **HDL** (beneficial) **cholesterol,** *foster* **arteriosclerosis,** and *increase* the risk of **coronary heart disease.**[109, 110] However, their effect is *not* as *injurious* as the **saturated fat** in milk, **cheese, egg's yolk, meat,** and **sausage.**[111]

  Regular consumption of trans fatty acids has also been related to breast cancer in postmenopausal women.[112]

Avoiding Constipation

Constipation is defined as *difficulty in defecation*. It is accompanied by:

- Expulsion of a small amount of hard feces,
- Reduction in defecation to less than three or four times a week.

Avoiding constipation is **essential** to enjoying good health.

1. Drink Enough Water

If the body is not properly hydrated, the large intestine extracts water from the feces. This dries them and makes them difficult to expel.

2. Eat a Proper Diet

Avoiding constipation requires a proper diet, increasing the intake of fiber. The foods that contribute most to constipation prevention are the following:

- **Fresh fruits** (except quince, persimmon, pomegranate, and loquat, which are astringents). **Dried fruits** such as prunes and raisins are also effective.
- **Vegetables**
- **Whole grains** and products made from them such as whole grain bread and pasta.

A daily diet consisting *primarily* of **milk, fish, meat,** and their derivatives **fosters** constipation.

3. Consume Enough Fiber

Plant-based foods are the only ones that contain the fiber necessary to, among other things, move the feces normally through the intestine.

The following page describes how to increase fiber consumption.

4. Educate the bowel

Laxatives (natural vegetable fiber and pharmaceutical preparations), enemas, glycerin suppositories, and other remedies may relieve an acute case, but not chronic constipation.

However, persistent functional constipation is not cured by these measures, which only provide temporary relief.

Avoiding constipation requires the learning of good toilet habits **from childhood** and educating the bowel.

- **Do not ignore** the physiological need to defecate.
- Try to evacuate at the **same** time of the day.
- Perform some type of **physical exercise.** These habits, *together* with a **proper diet,** are the **best** way to *avoid* constipation.

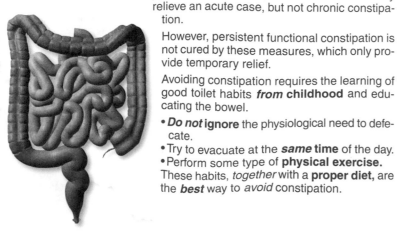

It is a Symptom

Constipation is a very common symptom, and is usually attributable to **functional disorders** or an **inadequate diet.** However, it may be the **early manifestation** of an intestinal tumor as **colon cancer, or other serious diseases.**

Constipation that appears **without an evident cause** or that **persists** should **always** be diagnosed by a **physician.**

How To Increase Fiber Intake

Fiber is a component of plant-based foods that has the following characteristics:

- It is **necessary** for proper intestinal function.
- It is **not digested nor** does it **pass** to the **bloodstream.** It remains in the intestine and forms part of the feces.
- It **retains water,** increasing fecal volume.
- Although it is not acted on by digestive enzymes, as are other carbohydrates, proteins and fats, it is partially fermented by bacterial flora in the colon. This results in various intestinal **gases.**
- Its consumption (at least 25 g daily for adults) contributes to the **prevention** of various diseases such as:
  - **Constipation**
  - **Diverticulosis**
  - **Colon cancer**
  - Excess **cholesterol** and **diabetes**.

Increase the Consumption of Legumes and Vegetables

Vegetables such as onions, asparagus, leeks, cabbage, as well as legumes contain **oligosaccharides,** a special type of **fiber** that is different from the cellulose that forms grain bran.

These oligosaccharides are metabolized by bacteria in the intestine, creating more or less bothersome but **innocuous** intestinal **gases.** In spite of the small inconvenience created by the gas, oligosaccharides provide various health benefits:[113]

- They *increase* the population of beneficial **bifidobacteria** in the intestinal flora.
- They *prevent* **constipation** by increasing the intensity of the intestine's **peristaltic action.**
- They *protect* against **colon cancer.**
- They *reduce* **cholesterol** levels.

Consume Bran or Other Fiber-rich Supplements

The *ideal* is to consume them in their **natural** state, forming part of grains or whole grain bread. However, it can be consumed as a supplement as long as no more than **30 g** are used daily. This amount of bran provides almost **13 g** of **pure fiber.**

Each gram of bran increases the weight of the feces by 2-3 grams since it retains 2-3 times its weight in water.

Flaxseed, glucomannan, and **agar-agar**, in addition to **bran**, are some of the most used high-fiber dietary supplements.

Eat Whole-grain Bread instead of White Bread

Whole-grain bread contains approximately three times the fiber of white bread.

Eat Fruit with all of its Pulp instead of Drinking Fruit Juice

Fruit juice contains virtually no fiber since it is found in the pulp.

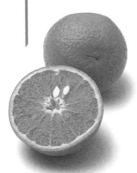

A breakfast of whole grains or whole-grain bread, with a few prunes and two pieces of fresh fruit can provide the 25 g of fiber that are needed daily.

A breakfast like this makes preventing constipation easy.

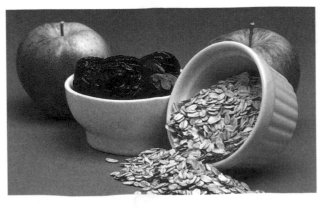

Update for Diabetics

Classic Diet for Diabetics

Until recently, diabetics were prescribed a diet

- Low in all types of carbohydrates
- Rich in proteins and fats

The use of whole grains, legumes, and fruits was discouraged because of their complex hydrocarbon (starch) and sugar content, which were transformed into glucose during digestion.

This carbohydrate-poor diet seemed the most logical for diabetics, and apparently allowed good blood-glucose level control. Nevertheless, it has been shown that diabetics eating this type of diet have a higher incidence of arteriosclerosis and cardiovascular disease, including heart attack.

*Excess **fat** and **protein,*** which *promotes **arteriosclerosis,*** combined with a lack of grains, legumes, and antioxidant fruits explain the *long-term* **harm done** by this type of diet.

■ ■ ■

Today's Diabetic Diet

Dietetic treatment of diabetics is constantly overcoming the old taboos concerning the drawbacks of carbohydrates. Today's dietary recommendation is:

1. *Rich* in **complex carbohydrates** (starch).
2. *Rich* in **fiber.**

3. *Low* in **fat,** particularly saturated animal fat.[115]

4. *Low* in **sugar.**

This approach provides *better results* in **controlling glycemia, preventing complications,** and **improving longevity** of diabetics.

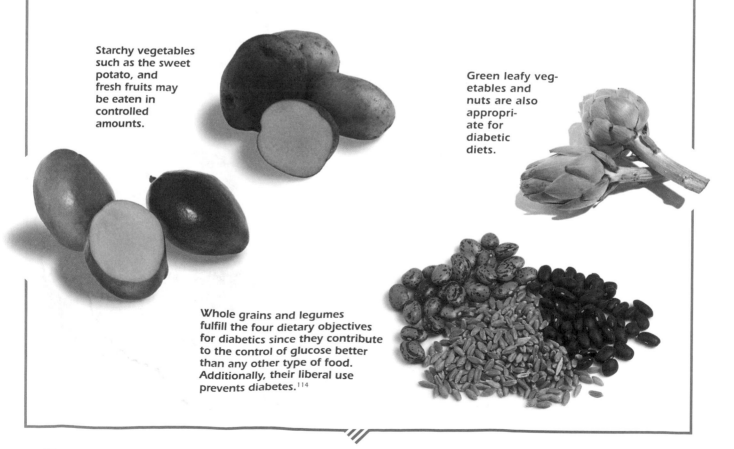

Starchy vegetables such as the sweet potato, and fresh fruits may be eaten in controlled amounts.

Green leafy vegetables and nuts are also appropriate for diabetic diets.

Whole grains and legumes fulfill the four dietary objectives for diabetics since they contribute to the control of glucose better than any other type of food. Additionally, their liberal use prevents diabetes.[114]

Healthful Foods Pyramid

The relative amount of each food group that should be consumed daily is represented by the size of each section of the pyramid.

The lower (closer to the base) a food group is situated, the more important it is to a healthful diet.

This food pyramid has been adapted from the one provided in 1995 by the US Department of Health and Human Services and the Department of Agriculture, published in the fourth edition of 'Nutrition and your Health: Dietary Guidelines for Americans.'

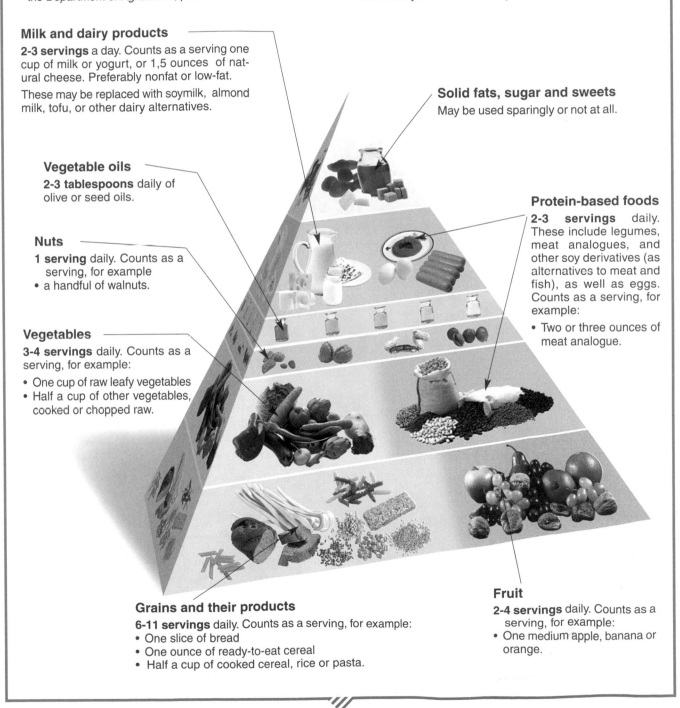

Milk and dairy products

2-3 servings a day. Counts as a serving one cup of milk or yogurt, or 1,5 ounces of natural cheese. Preferably nonfat or low-fat.

These may be replaced with soymilk, almond milk, tofu, or other dairy alternatives.

Solid fats, sugar and sweets

May be used sparingly or not at all.

Vegetable oils

2-3 tablespoons daily of olive or seed oils.

Protein-based foods

2-3 servings daily. These include legumes, meat analogues, and other soy derivatives (as alternatives to meat and fish), as well as eggs. Counts as a serving, for example:

- Two or three ounces of meat analogue.

Nuts

1 serving daily. Counts as a serving, for example
- a handful of walnuts.

Vegetables

3-4 servings daily. Counts as a serving, for example:

- One cup of raw leafy vegetables
- Half a cup of other vegetables, cooked or chopped raw.

Grains and their products

6-11 servings daily. Counts as a serving, for example:
- One slice of bread
- One ounce of ready-to-eat cereal
- Half a cup of cooked cereal, rice or pasta.

Fruit

2-4 servings daily. Counts as a serving, for example:
- One medium apple, banana or orange.

Reduce Total Caloric Intake

For a diet to be effective for losing weight, it must supply *fewer calories* than those the *body burns.*

This is confirmed by a study by the University of Geneva (Switzerland) according to which the fewer calories a diet provides, the greater the weight loss.[117]

Maintain a Balanced Proportion of the Sources of Calories

The calories consumed in a weight-loss diet should *not* be concentrated *only* on *proteins* or *fats* as some propose.

Ideally, the **caloric** intake in a healthy weight-loss diet should be balanced among the **three food energy** *sources* as illustrated in the graph below.

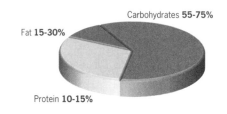

Carbohydrates **55-75%**
Fat **15-30%**
Protein **10-15%**

The **advantages** of a diet that maintains this optimal balance of calories from carbohydrates, fats, and proteins are:

• It does *not* produce **metabolic imbalances** seen when one nutrient, carbohydrates, for example, is reduced or eliminated.

• It can be followed for **long periods** with no ill effects.

• It provides a *more* **long-lasting effect.**

Choose Satiating Foods

These tend to be *fiber-rich.* As it retains water, fiber increases in volume in the stomach and produces a sense of satiety.

Foods that produce this sensation are **vegetables** in general, **seaweed, sweet potato,** and some **fruits,** such as cherries.

Choose Low-energy-producing Foods

Increase consumption of foods supplying few calories in proportion to their weight such as **vegetables** and **fruits**.

High-energy-producing foods, those with higher concentrations of calories, may be classified in two groups:

• **Healthful,** such as **oils** (olive, seed oils), oil-bearing **nuts,** and **dried fruit** may be eaten in *small, measured amounts.*

• **Unhealthful,** such as pastries, chocolate, fried foods, sausages, and patés should be *completely avoided.*

Learn Healthful Dietary Habits

• **Eat slowly,** chewing all foods carefully. It is a proven fact that eating in this way reduces the amount of food consumed, thus fewer calories.

• *Do not* eat between meals.

• *Avoid* **anxiety** and **worry** at mealtime, since this unconsciously leads to greater consumption.

• Make **breakfast** and **lunch** the *primary meals* of the day, *eliminating* supper or *reducing* it to a salad or a little fruit.

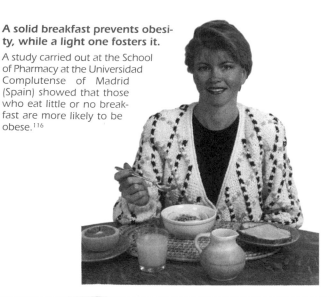

A solid breakfast prevents obesity, while a light one fosters it.

A study carried out at the School of Pharmacy at the Universidad Complutense of Madrid (Spain) showed that those who eat little or no breakfast are more likely to be obese.[116]

Weight Gain

Cherries or Pastry?

Calories are not the only important thing

One-half kilo of **cherries** (about 1 pound) supplies **360 kcal,** approximately the same as **100 g** (about 3.5 ounces) of chocolate **pastry.**

Eating the same number of calories, the pastry fosters obesity, while the cherries prevent it.

In a weight-loss diet, not only is the **number** of calories important, but their **source,** as well. Equal amounts of calories from grains, vegetables, legumes, and fruits are less fattening than sweets, refined baked goods, sausages, and patés.

One reason cherries help prevent obesity is that they take longer to eat. In contrast, concentrated foods eaten rapidly tend to increase caloric intake.

1/2 Kilo of Cherries

• **Is** eaten **slowly** (about 10 minutes).

• Produces a feeling of **satiety.**

• Supplies rapidly absorbed simple **sugars,** but since they are combined with **fiber,** they are absorbed more **slowly** than if they were part of a pastry.

• Contains **B** group **vitamins,** which facilitate the metabolism of sugars. Consequently, they are utilized more easily than if they were part of a pastry.

One Hundred Grams of Pastry

• Are eaten **rapidly** (a minute or less).

• Are **not filling,** so one continues eating.

• Contain **saturated fats** and **refined carbohydrates,** which become **fatty deposits** in the body unless intense physical exercise is done to burn them.

The concept that carbohydrates are "fattening" and therefore have no place in a weight loss diet must be discarded.

Whole grain cereals and breads, legumes, and fruits supply carbohydrates that can be safely eaten in controlled amounts in a healthful weight loss diet.

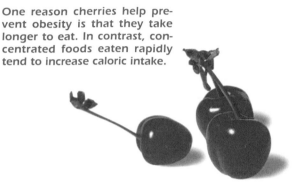

Diabetics, like the obese, must become accustomed to eating controlled and weighed portions of each food, with the objective of not exceeding the total daily allowance and maintaining the balance among nutrients.

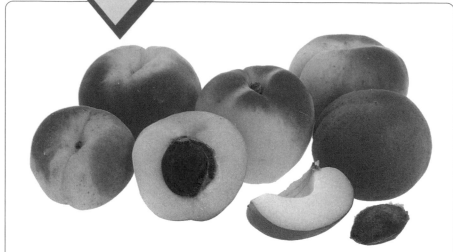

Apricot

Gives sparkle and beauty to the eyes

THE APRICOT tree is famous for being one of the most traveled trees known. Its origin is in the north of China, where it is still found wild.

It was taken to Greece by Alexander the Great on the return from his conquests in India. From Greece it passed to Rome, from where its cultivation spread throughout the Mediterranean region. In the 18th century it was taken to North America, where it acclimated to California and states along the Mississippi River. And its long journey does not end here. American astronauts took it to the moon on one of their space journeys.

Synonym: *Apricock;*
French: *Abricot;*
Spanish: *Albaricoque, damasco;*
German: *Aprikose.*

Description: *Fruit of the apricot tree ('Prunus armeniaca' L.) from the botanical family Rosaceae. The tree may reach a height of ten meters.*

Habitat: *Originally from central Asia. The apricot has acclimated to temperate climates in Europe and America.*

Apricots are usually eaten with the skin. Because of this, the ideal is to eat those grown organically to avoid ingesting chemical products such as pesticides that impregnate the skin and are difficult to remove even by thorough washing.

APRICOT
Composition
per 100 g of raw edible portion

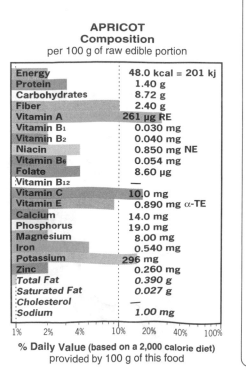

Energy	48.0 kcal = 201 kj
Protein	1.40 g
Carbohydrates	8.72 g
Fiber	2.40 g
Vitamin A	261 µg RE
Vitamin B₁	0.030 mg
Vitamin B₂	0.040 mg
Niacin	0.850 mg NE
Vitamin B₆	0.054 mg
Folate	8.60 µg
Vitamin B₁₂	—
Vitamin C	10.0 mg
Vitamin E	0.890 mg α-TE
Calcium	14.0 mg
Phosphorus	19.0 mg
Magnesium	8.00 mg
Iron	0.540 mg
Potassium	296 mg
Zinc	0.260 mg
Total Fat	*0.390 g*
Saturated Fat	*0.027 g*
Cholesterol	—
Sodium	*1.00 mg*

1% 2% 4% 10% 20% 40% 100%

% Daily Value (based on a 2,000 calorie diet)
provided by 100 g of this food

APRICOT

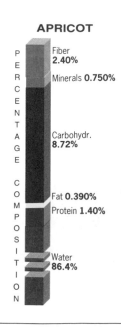

PERCENTAGE COMPOSITION

Fiber 2.40%
Minerals 0.750%
Carbohydr. 8.72%
Fat 0.390%
Protein 1.40%
Water 86.4%

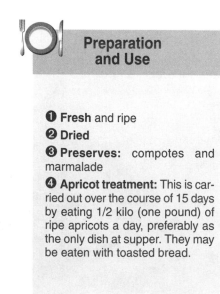

Preparation and Use

❶ **Fresh** and ripe

❷ **Dried**

❸ **Preserves:** compotes and marmalade

❹ **Apricot treatment:** This is carried out over the course of 15 days by eating 1/2 kilo (one pound) of ripe apricots a day, preferably as the only dish at supper. They may be eaten with toasted bread.

Its attractive orange color, its pleasant aroma, and its delicious sweetness have made the apricot one of the favorite fruits of the summer season. Dried apricots and marmalade allow this pleasure to last through the winter, as well.

PROPERTIES AND INDICATIONS: The fact that the apricot has a low calorie content (about 48 kcal/100 g) makes it an excellent part of **weight-loss diets.** It has an **alkalizing** effect because of its richness in alkaline mineral salts. It is particularly noted for its *low sodium content* and its *high levels of potassium.* It contains various trace elements of great physiological importance, such as manganese, fluorine, cobalt, and boron. It is rich in sugars (*fructose* and *glucose*).

Dried apricots are an important source of **protein** (up to 5%). They also are an important source of *iron,* one of their principal minerals.

However, the most important component of apricots, whether fresh or dried, is beta-carotene or **provitamin A.** This component provides most of its therapeutic value, which are the following:

• **Diseases of the eye:** Consumption of apricots maintains vision in good condition and gives the sparkle and beauty to the eyes that are characteristic of good health. This is not due exclusively to the action of provitamin A, but also to the combined action of other vitamins and minerals that accompany it.

Apricots are recommended in cases of **conjunctival dryness, chronic irritation** or **itching** of the conjunctiva, **loss of visual acuity** due to retinal atrophy, and **night blindness.**

The *best results* are obtained by following an **apricot treatment** regime [❹].

• **Anemia** (due to lack of iron): The iron content of fresh apricots is not significant, whereas it is in the dried fruit [❷]. For reasons that are not well understood, the *results* achieved through their use in the treatment of anemia are far superior to those that would be expected given their low proportion of iron. This may be because of the presence of other substances in apricots that facilitate the absorption of iron.

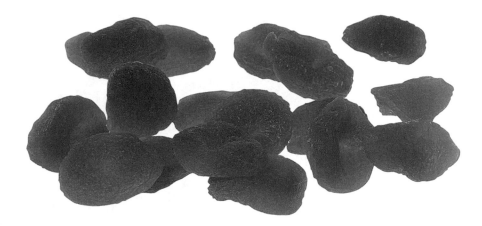

Besides being delicious, dried apricots are a good source of provitamin A because of their richness in beta-carotene.

They ought to have been dried and preserved naturally without any additives or preservatives (usually sulfites), as the latter can cause various allergic reactions (like asthma attacks) in sensitized persons.

Jean Valnet, an outstanding French physician who dedicated his life to the study of phytotherapy and diet therapy, quotes previous experiences of *Leclerc* stating that it has been experimentally proven that apricot treatment [❹] provides results similar to those of beef liver in cases of anemia due to loss of blood.[118]

The amounts of provitamin A and iron found in apricots are actually quite small compared to the large doses that pharmaceutical preparations may contain. In spite of this, the results obtained from regular consumption of this fruit are superior to those to be expected from their content of *iron* and *provitamin A.*

This is one of the most surprising facts in nutrition science. It has been scientifically explained only in the last few years. The happy *combination* of vitamins, minerals, and other chemical substances present in natural foods enhances their *action.* The results obtained by the use of natural whole foods are superior to those obtained by their isolated and purified components as found in pharmaceutical preparations.

• **Disorders of the skin and mucosa,** due to their content of provitamin A. Apricots increase resistance to infections. They are recommended for chronic **pharyngitis, sinusitis,** and **eczema.**

• **Nervous disorders:** Dr. *Valnet* points out the apricot's properties of maintaining equilibrium within the nervous system and recommends it in cases **of asthenia, depression, nervousness,** and **lack of appetite.** These effects are attributed to the apricot's richness in **trace elements.**

• **Digestive disorders:** *Fresh,* ripe apricots are slightly **astringent [❶],** while dried apricots are **laxative [❷].**

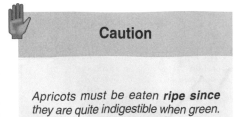

Caution

Apricots must be eaten **ripe since** they are quite indigestible when green.

The industrial drying process used for apricots frequently includes **sulfites** as preservatives. This additive can provoke **asthma attacks** in allergic individuals.

| Lactuca sativa L. | pH↑ | | | | | | | |

Lettuce

Calms the nerves and satisfies the stomach

THE ANCIENT Romans ate lettuce at night as a sleep aid after overeating at supper. Today the stressed inhabitants of modern cities can benefit from this effect of lettuce *not after*, but rather *in place of a big supper.*

Lettuce as a first or only dish for supper is ideal for those requiring its sedative effect or those seeking a remedy for obesity. In this way its mild sedative effect and its ability to satisfy the appetite are maximized. Naturally, those who are under the stress of a weight-loss diet need to retire early, so that when the sense of satiety has passed in two or three hours he or she is asleep.

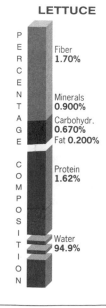

Scientific synonym: *Lactuca virosa* L.

Synonyms: *Celtuce, Cos, Garden lettuce, [Green] romaine lettuce;*
French: *Laitue;* **Spanish:** *Lechuga;*
German: *Kopfsalat.*

Description: *Leaves of the lettuce plant 'Lactuca sativa', of the botanical family Compositae. There are varieties with straight leaves and others with curly ones, and their color varies from green to purple red.*

Habitat: *Originally from Asia Minor, its cultivation extended in antiquity throughout the Roman Empire. It is presently grown in the open air in temperate areas throughout the world, as well as in green houses.*

Roman lettuce grown in the open air, whose composition appears to the left, is much richer in provitamin A, folates and iron than other varieties.

Lettuce grown in green houses is whiter but less nutritious, and they also contain more nitrates because of the usage of chemical fertilizers.

LETTUCE
Composition
per 100 g of raw edible portion

Energy	16.0 kcal = 67.0 kj
Protein	1.62 g
Carbohydrates	0.670 g
Fiber	1.70 g
Vitamin A	260 µg RE
Vitamin B₁	0.100 mg
Vitamin B₂	0.100 mg
Niacin	0.700 mg NE
Vitamin B₆	0.047 mg
Folate	136 µg
Vitamin B₁₂	—
Vitamin C	24.0 mg
Vitamin E	0.440 mg α-TE
Calcium	36.0 mg
Phosphorus	45.0 mg
Magnesium	6.00 mg
Iron	1.10 mg
Potassium	290 mg
Zinc	0.250 mg
Total Fat	0.200 g
Saturated Fat	0.026 g
Cholesterol	—
Sodium	8.00 mg

1%   2%   4%   10%   20%   40%   100%

% Daily Value (based on a 2,000 calorie diet) provided by 100 g of this food

LETTUCE

PERCENTAGE COMPOSITION

Fiber
1.70%

Minerals
0.900%
Carbohydr.
0.670%
Fat **0.200%**

Protein
1.62%

Water
94.9%

Preparation and Use

❶ **Raw:** This is best way to enjoy its freshness and pleasant taste. It is dressed with a little oil (preferably olive oil) and a few drops of lemon juice. Green leaves are much more nutritious than the white ones on the inside.

❷ **Cooked:** The toughest leaves can be cooked like any other green.

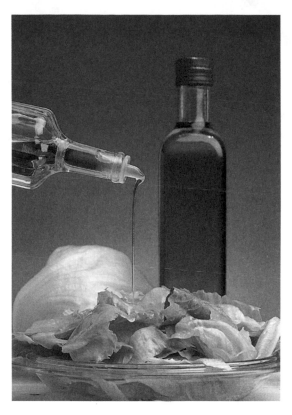

Having a good dish of lettuce, properly dressed with oil and lemon, eases digestion and helps to induce sleep, besides producing a remarkable sensation of satiety.

PROPERTIES AND INDICATIONS: Lettuce is one of the foods richest in *water* (94.9%). However, the relatively high level of proteins (1.62%) that it provides is surprising. This is only slightly less than the potato (2.07%). These are incomplete proteins, since the essential amino acid methionine is present in insufficient quantities. However, combining lettuce with a plate of legumes (preferably at the same meal), a supplementation takes place between the proteins of both foods and the body obtains all of the amino acids needed in the proper proportion.

Lettuce is a very poor source of carbohydrates (0.67%) and fat (0.2%), which explains its low energetic contribution. The nutritional and therapeutic value of lettuce is based on the following components:

✓ *Provitamin A:* 100 g of lettuce provides 260 µg RE (micrograms of retinol equivalents), which represents a quarter of the daily requirement of this provitamin. The white leaves in the center contain much less provitamin A in the form of *beta-carotene.*

✓ *B group vitamins:* Lettuce is quite rich in vitamin B_1 (0.1 mg/100 g) and B_2 (0.1 mg/100 g), and, above all, *folates* (135.7 µg/100 g).

✓ *Vitamin C:* The concentration of this vitamin in lettuce is 24 mg/100 g, a little less than half that of the orange or lemon.

✓ *Minerals:* Lettuce is noted for its potassium (290 mg/100 g) and iron (1.1 mg/100 g) content. It has significant amounts of calcium, phosphorous, and magnesium, as well as the trace elements zinc, copper, and manganese. These minerals form alkalizing salts, making lettuce a good **antacid** in the stomach as well as in the blood.

✓ *Vegetable fiber* (1.7%) that contributes a mild laxative effect.

✓ *Sedative and sleep-inducing substances,* the same as found in the *latex* of wild lettuce[119] (lactucarium), but in much lower proportion. These substances are chemically similar to those from opium, but they are completely lacking in toxicity and addictive properties.

Because of this composition, lettuce has the following properties: sedative, sleep inducing, aperitif, alkalizer, and remineralizer. It is indicated for the following conditions:

• **Functional disorders of the nervous system,** such as nervousness, stress or psychological tension, or anxiety. Regular lettuce consumption produces a mild, and sometimes imperceptible sedative effect, while providing necessary B vitamins for nervous system stability.

• **Insomnia:** A large supper consisting of *only lettuce* is recommended at *night* for insomnia.

• **Digestive disorders:** When eaten *before a meal*, lettuce tones the stomach and facilitates digestion.

• **Constipation:** Lettuce facilitates intestinal function because of its excellent digestibility and *fiber* content.

• **Obesity:** Lettuce produces a great sense of satiety, but provides few calories. At the same time, it helps relieve nervousness and anxiety regarding food that often accompanies obesity. A large plate of lettuce significantly reduces the appetite in addition to providing a considerable amount of vitamins and minerals.

• **Diabetes:** Lettuce is *very low* in **carbohydrates**; therefore, diabetics can eat it limited only by the appetite.

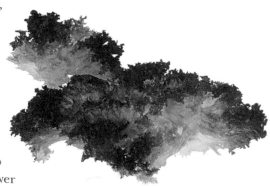

Walnut

Provides energy to the heart

EVEN THOUGH it is believed that the walnut originated in Central Asia, it has adapted very well to the countries surrounding the Mediterranean. It may be said that for millennia the walnut has formed part of the Mediterranean diet, which is praised for its beneficial effects on health in general and on the heart in particular.

Synonyms: *Persian walnut, Heartnut;*
French: *Noix;* **Spanish:** *Nuez;*
German: *Walnuß.*

Description: *the walnut is the seed of the fruit of the walnut tree ('Juglans regia' L.), a tree of the botanical family Juglandaceae that grows to a height of 20 meters. The fruit is a drupe, whose fleshy portion (pericarp and mesocarp) is greenish; the seed or endocarp is woody and hard, but it contains a very nutritious dicotyledonous seed: the walnut.*

Habitat: *Walnuts require a temperate, somewhat cool climate. They grow well in valleys and other places protected from freezing in winter. Today their cultivation has extended throughout the temperate regions of the world, particularly Europe, Asia, and North America.*

Walnuts are a highly concentrated food containing high levels of essential fatty acids, vitamin B$_6$ and trace elements such as zinc, copper, and manganese.

WALNUT
Composition
per 100 g of raw edible portion

Energy	642 kcal = 2,686 kj
Protein	14.3 g
Carbohydrates	13.5 g
Fiber	4.80 g
Vitamin A	12.0 µg RE
Vitamin B$_1$	0.382 mg
Vitamin B$_2$	0.148 mg
Niacin	4.19 mg NE
Vitamin B$_6$	0.558 mg
Folate	66.0 µg
Vitamin B$_{12}$	—
Vitamin C	3.20 mg
Vitamin E	2.62 mg α-TE
Calcium	94.0 mg
Phosphorus	317 mg
Magnesium	169 mg
Iron	2.44 mg
Potassium	502 mg
Zinc	2.73 mg
Total Fat	61.9 g
Saturated Fat	5.59 g
Cholesterol	—
Sodium	10.0 mg

1%   2%   4%   10%   20%   40%   100%

% Daily Value (based on a 2,000 calorie diet) provided by 100 g of this food

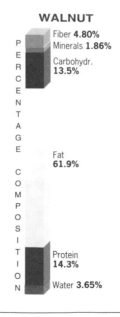

Saturated **5.59 g**
Monounsat. **14.2 g**
Polyunsat. **39.1 g**

Percentage distribution of **fatty acids**

WALNUT

P E R C E N T A G E   C O M P O S I T I O N

Fiber 4.80%
Minerals 1.86%
Carbohydr. 13.5%
Fat 61.9%
Protein 14.3%
Water 3.65%

Preparation and Use

❶ **Raw and whole:** Raw walnuts must be chewed very well. If they are indigestible, elimination of the thin yellow skin may help.

❷ **Ground:** Ground walnuts are easily assimilated by those with chewing difficulty.

❸ **Cooked:** A great variety of delicious vegetarian dishes can be made from walnuts including meat analogues, "meat" balls, and many others.

❹ **Walnut oil:** This is very flavorful and nutritious, but is seldom available commercially because it becomes rancid very easily.

During the 16th century Spanish sailors took the walnut to North America. It acclimated particularly well in California, one of the world's largest producers of these nuts. California walnuts are large and attractive, although gourmets still prefer the flavor of the smaller and wrinkled nuts from the old Mediterranean trees.

PROPERTIES AND INDICATIONS: The walnut is, together with other oil-bearing nuts, one of the *most concentrated* food sources of nutrients provided by nature. Together with the Brazil nut, it is the nut with the *highest caloric* content (642 kcal/100 g), due to its high fat content (oil). These are the characteristics of the walnut's nutrients:

✓ *Fats:* They fats are formed *primarily* of **unsaturated fatty acids,** with a preponderance of *polyunsaturated,* in addition to *lecithin.*

✓ *Carbohydrates:* The walnut is the lowest of any oil-bearing nut in this nutrient (13.5%). Because of this, walnuts are well tolerated by diabetics.

✓ *Proteins:* Walnuts contain up to 14.3% of high quality protein, more than peanuts, and about the same as almonds. They are somewhat deficient in the essential amino acid methionine, which is solved by *combining* them with **whole grains** (wheat, oats, rice, etc.), which are very rich in *methionine.*

✓ *Vitamins:* Walnuts are a good source of vitamins B_1, B_2, B_3 (niacin), and particularly B_6. They are relatively poor in vitamins A and C.

✓ *Minerals:* Walnuts are rich in *phosphorous* and *potassium,* while they are low in *sodium,* which promotes cardiovascular health.

With this rich and varied nutritional composition, walnuts have the following therapeutic applications:

• **Coronary disease:** Walnuts are heart-friendly for these three reasons, and should be *included regularly* in the diets of those suffering from **heart failure** for any reason, **angina,** or **heart attack** *risk*. Their consumption is particularly recommended for those who have suffered a myocardial infarction and are in rehabilitation.

• **Elevated cholesterol:** Up until not long ago the consumption of oil-bearing nuts, and walnuts in particular, was discouraged for those with elevated cholesterol levels. However, investigations conducted by Dr. Joan Sabaté at Loma Linda University (California), demonstrate[120] that daily consumption of 80 g of walnuts for two months, reduces the level of LDL (harmful) by 16%.

This blood cholesterol-lowering action, with its positive effect on arteriosclerosis results when walnuts *replace* other foods such as **margarine, butter,** or **sausage.** This *helps avoid* the fattening mistakenly attributed to nuts.

• **Disorders of the nervous system:** Walnuts are highly recommended for neurological disorders in general because of their *richness* in **essential fatty** acids directly involved in the metabolism of the neurons, and in *lecithin, phosphorous,* and *vitamin B_6.*

Because they improve mental performance and restore tone and balance to the nervous system, they should form a part of the diets of **students** and **knowledge workers.** Those suffering from **irritability, depression, stress,** or **nervous exhaustion** should eat at least a good handful of walnuts a day, preferably at breakfast.

• Sexual disorders and sterility: one of the many functions of *linoleic* and linolenic acids, which are so abundant in walnuts, is to serve as the base for the synthesis of *PROSTAGLANDINS.* These substances perform various functions, such as mediating **inflammatory reactions.** It is also believed that they are involved in the physiological phenomena associated with sexual response; in fact, **semen** is very rich in *prostaglandins.*

Whether because of this, their vitamin B_1 and B_6 content, or because of the walnut's richness in trace elements, which facilitate many chemical reactions within the cells, it is certain that walnut consumption has a positive effect on sexual performance: it *increases* a **man's potency** and improves a *woman's* **sexual response.**

It cannot be said that walnuts are an aphrodisiac in the strict sense of the word since walnuts do not really increase sexual desire, but they do facilitate the complex physiological reactions produced during sexual activity in both men and women.

• **Diabetes:** Because of their low carbohydrate content and high nutritional value, walnuts are one of the foods best tolerated by diabetics.

• **Increase in nutritional needs:** because of their high caloric and nutritive value, eating walnuts is highly recommended for situations in which the body is involved in extraordinary effort: **athletes, students** preparing for examinations, **pregnant** or **nursing** women, convalescence from a debilitating disease, and physical **stress** in general.

Walnuts Against Heart Attack

A study conducted in California known as the Adventist Health Study, analyzed the dietary habits of more than 25,000 Seventh-day Adventist, Christians universally recognized for their healthy lifestyle.

The results showed that heart attack risk among Adventists is considerably lower than that of the general population.

Additionally, those that ate walnuts five or more times a week, had an even lower risk of heart attack: approximately half of the Adventists in the study ate walnuts at least once a week.[139]

Chickpea

Just the thing for modern men and women

IN INDIA, where a large part of the population follows a primarily vegetarian diet, chickpeas are a main protein source.

In the same way, chickpeas have been a fundamental ingredient in the traditional diets of the peoples living along the coasts of the Mediterranean.

Because of this, perhaps, chickpeas have been considered a "food of the poor" by "modern, developed" city-dwellers. However, it is precisely these individuals, menaced by the diseases of civilization (arteriosclerosis, heart attack, stress, etc.), that need a good plate of chickpeas.

PROPERTIES AND INDICATIONS: The noteworthy therapeutic properties of the chickpea make this humble legume a dietary food ideal for modern men and women: they help *reduce* **cholesterol** and avoid **constipation** while *strengthening* the **nervous system.**

Additionally, the chickpea is nourishing and balanced as it contains a great deal of energy (364 kcal/100 g). It is a good source of the most important nutrients except vitamin B12 (which is true of all plant-based foods). Even provitamin A and vitamins C and E are present, but only in small amounts. The remaining nutrients are well represented in the chickpea:

✓ *Proteins:* Chickpeas provide a significant amount (19.3%), equal or superior to **meat** and **eggs** but less than other protein-rich legumes such as soy, lentils, or beans. These are *complete proteins* that contain all of the amino acids (essential and nonessential) with the exception of the sulfu-

Synonyms: *Ceci, Garbanzo [bean], Bengal gram, Calvance pea, Chick pea, Dwarf pea, Gram pea, Yellow gram;*
French: *Pois chiche;*
Spanish: *Garbanzo, chícharo;*
German: *Kichererbse.*

Description: *The seed of the chickpea plant ('Cicer arietinum' L.), of the botanical family Leguminosae. Its fruit is an ovoid legume containing two seeds, chickpeas.*

Habitat: *Chickpeas are very resistant to drought, as well as to extremes of heat and cold. India controls 70% of the world chickpea production. Other producing countries are Mexico, Turkey, and Mediterranean countries.*

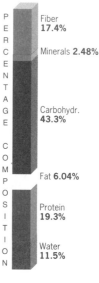

PERCENTAGE COMPOSITION
- Fiber **17.4%**
- Minerals **2.48%**
- Carbohydr. **43.3%**
- Fat **6.04%**
- Protein **19.3%**
- Water **11.5%**

CHICKPEA Composition
per 100 g of raw edible portion

Energy	364 kcal = 1,525 kj
Protein	19.3 g
Carbohydrates	43.3 g
Fiber	17.4 g
Vitamin A	7.00 µg RE
Vitamin B1	0.477 mg
Vitamin B2	0.212 mg
Niacin	4.62 mg NE
Vitamin B6	0.535 mg
Folate	557 µg
Vitamin B12	—
Vitamin C	4.00 mg
Vitamin E	0.820 mg α-TE
Calcium	105 mg
Phosphorus	366 mg
Magnesium	115 mg
Iron	6.24 mg
Potassium	875 mg
Zinc	3.43 mg
Total Fat	6.04 g
Saturated Fat	0.626 g
Cholesterol	—
Sodium	24.0 mg

1% 2% 4% 10% 20% 40% 100% 200% 500%
% Daily Value (based on a 2,000 calorie diet) provided by 100 g of this food

Preparation and Use

❶ **Cooked:** This is the most common manner of preparing and eating chickpeas in the West. They can be added to soups and stews. They combine very well with rice dishes.

❷ **Oven toasted or fried:** When prepared in this way they are somewhat indigestible since a part of the starch becomes resistant to gastric juices.[19]

❸ **Chickpea flour:** This is widely used in India to make a variety of culinary items such as *falafel.*

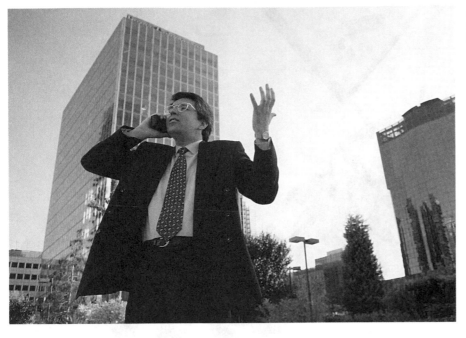

Although it has been somewhat forgotten today, chickpeas are a perfect choice for this generation:

- They reduce cholesterol levels,
- They prevent constipation,
- They strengthen the nervous system thanks to their richness in B group vitamins.

rated amino acid *methionine,* which is not found in an optimal proportion.

This protein deficiency, which is true of all legumes in general, has been exaggerated by some nutritional specialists. They have not considered that any grain, such as wheat or rice that is eaten with chickpeas *more than compensates* for its relative lack of methionine. The legume-grain combination produces a protein of excellent biological quality.[122]

✓ *Carbohydrates:* Chickpeas are very rich in carbohydrates (43.3%), starch being predominant. Starch is transformed slowly to glucose during digestion, but it must be well chewed and salivated.

✓ *Fat:* Chickpeas are 6.04% fat. This is considerably more than lentils or beans, but less than soy. Most of these fats are *polyunsaturated.*

✓ *Vitamins:* B group vitamins are the most abundant in chickpeas. One hundred grams of chickpeas provide 0.477 mg of vitamin B_1, which represents a third of the daily need for this vitamin. Chickpeas are also a good source of vitamins B_2 and B_6. *Folates,* which are also involved in proper nervous system function and the reduction of heart attack risk, are *very abundant:* One hundred grams of chickpeas supply almost *triple* the RDA

(Recommended Dietary Allowance) of this nutrient.

✓ *Minerals:* The most noteworthy are *iron* (6.24 mg/100 g, almost *three times* that of **meat**), phosphorous (366 mg /100 g), potassium (875 mg /100 g), magnesium (115 mg/100 g), calcium (105 mg/100 mg), and *zinc* (3.43 mg /100 g).

Chickpeas are an ***almost* complete food** whose nutritional proportions are quite well balanced. For this reason, they can be used as the main dish of a meal, as is the case in a traditional Mediterranean diet. Eating chickpeas regularly is recommended in the following situations:

• **Increased cholesterol:** Chickpeas contain a moderate amount of high-quality (mono and polyunsaturated) fats (6.04%) that aid in lowering blood cholesterol level. Chickpeas' *fiber* also impedes the absorption of cholesterol from other foods in the intestine (chickpeas contain no cholesterol). Consequently, eating more chickpeas and fewer meat products reduces cholesterol levels and improves arterial health. Finally, eating chickpeas *prevents* **arteriosclerosis** in all of its manifestations, including heart attack.

• **Constipation:** The fiber in chickpeas naturally stimulates intestinal

peristaltic action thus moving the feces through the lower digestive tract.

• **Functional disorders of the nervous system** due to B vitamin deficiency, such as irritability, nervousness, and lack of concentration. Chickpeas are highly recommended for those suffering from **stress** or **depression.**

• **Pregnancy: For pregnant women** this legume is an ideal food because it is rich in *folates,* which prevent nervous system defects in the fetus. Additionally, chickpeas have a very *high content* of **proteins, iron,** and other *minerals.*

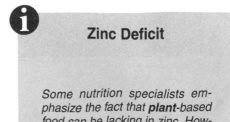

Zinc Deficit

*Some nutrition specialists emphasize the fact that **plant**-based food can be lacking in zinc. However, 100 g chickpeas contains more zinc (3.43 mg) than the same quantity of **meat** (2.97 mg). Chickpeas, the same as lentils and soy, are an excellent source of **zinc.***

Red beet

Its red juice combats anemia

THE BLOOD-RED color of beets gives a cheerful note to salads and potato dishes. Could it be that red beets truly contain blood?

Those who have passed blood-red urine or feces a few hours after eating beets might think so. What a fright! But it is not blood, but rather a pigment specific to this plant called **betacyanin.**

According to a study carried out at the University of Sheffield[123] (UK), red urine or feces after eating beets occurs in 10% to 14% of the population, and it is more frequent in individuals with iron deficiency or difficulty with intestinal absorption of iron. So if one is surprised by red elim-

French: Betterave;
Spanish: Remolacha, Remolacha de mesa, Remolacha colorada;
German: Rote Bete.

Description: *The tuberous root of the red beet ('Beta vulgaris' L. ssp. 'vulgaris' var. 'conditiva' Alef.), a herbaceous plant of the botanical family Chenopodiaceae.*

Habitat: *Beets are cultivated throughout Europe and North America. They adapt well to cold climates.*

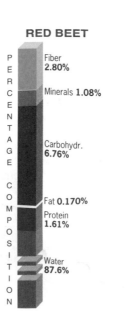

RED BEET

Fiber	2.80%
Minerals	1.08%
Carbohydr.	6.76%
Fat	0.170%
Protein	1.61%
Water	87.6%

PERCENTAGE COMPOSITION

RED BEET
Composition
per 100 g of raw edible portion

Energy	**43.0 kcal = 179 kj**
Protein	**1.61 g**
Carbohydrates	**6.76 g**
Fiber	**2.80 g**
Vitamin A	**4.00 µg RE**
Vitamin B$_1$	**0.031 mg**
Vitamin B$_2$	**0.040 mg**
Niacin	**0.651 mg NE**
Vitamin B$_6$	**0.067 mg**
Folate	**109 µg**
Vitamin B$_{12}$	**—**
Vitamin C	**4.90 mg**
Vitamin E	**0.300 mg α-TE**
Calcium	**16.0 mg**
Phosphorus	**40.0 mg**
Magnesium	**23.0 mg**
Iron	**0.800 mg**
Potassium	**325 mg**
Zinc	**0.350 mg**
Total Fat	*0.170 g*
Saturated Fat	*0.027 g*
Cholesterol	*—*
Sodium	*78.0 mg*

1%   2%   4%   10%   20%   40%   100%

% Daily Value (based on a 2,000 calorie diet)
provided by 100 g of this food

Preparation and Use

❶ **Fresh juice:** The flavor of beet juice is unpleasant and may be mixed with other juices or sweetened with honey to make it more palatable. No more than 50 to 100 ml should be drunk at a time to avoid indigestion.

❷ **Grated raw:** Beets prepared in this way may be dressed with lemon and oil.

❸ **Boiled:** Cooked beets are more digestible. They should be boiled for at least an hour. They are easier to peel if dipped in cold water while they are still hot.

ination, he or she should be grateful that this plant has warned of a possible lack of iron or digestive problems.

However, one should not worry excessively: Beets not only warn of the problem, but aid in its solution, thanks to their anti-anemic and regulating effects on the digestive system.

PROPERTIES AND INDICATIONS: Carbohydrates (sugars) such as saccharose and fructose are prominent in beets' composition. These can reach 10% of their weight. This makes the red beet one of the most sugar-rich vegetables, surpassed only by other varieties of beets (see box on this page). These are beets' most notable characteristics:

• **Anti-anemic:** The anti-anemic action of red beets is well known, and has been described by Doctor Schneider among others. Their iron content (1.80 mg/100 g) and vitamin C (30 mg/100 g) which facilitates the absorption of that mineral are quite modest and alone do not explain red beets' anti-anemic effect. It is probably some unidentified component that stimulates hematopoiesis (production of blood cells in the bone marrow).

Drinking 50 to 100 ml of *raw, freshly* prepared beet **juice (❶)** before meals

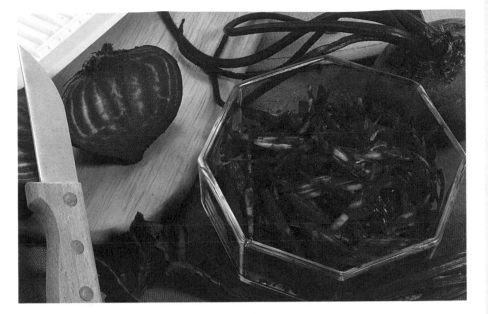

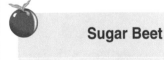

Sugar Beet

*The sugar beet is a botanical variety ('Beta vulgaris' L. ssp. 'vulgaris' var. 'altissima') that is **very rich** in **sugars** (saccharose), but is not appropriate for direct consumption.*

*The **juice** of the sugar beet contains up to 20% **saccharose**. Because of this, it is cultivated for industrial production of white sugar (saccharose).*

***French:** Betterave à sucre; **Spanish:** Remolacha azucarera; **German:** Zuckerrübe.*

twice a day provides the *greatest* **anti-anemic effect.** This is particularly indicated when the patient does not respond well to iron treatment, which is the case in anemia caused by low blood production in the bone marrow (hypoplastic anemia).

• **Alkalizer:** Beet's high levels of mineral salts, particularly *potassium, calcium,* and *magnesium,* explain their alkalizing effect on the blood. They are highly recommended in case of **gout,** increase in **uric acid** levels in the blood, and a **high-fat low vegetable diet.**

• **Hypolipidemic:** The beet root contains considerable vegetable fiber, which has the property of facilitating intestinal action and, above all, decreasing blood cholesterol level by reducing the amount absorbed in the intestine. A University of Minnesota[125] (USA) study showed that 30 mg of beet fiber a day during three weeks lowered total cholesterol by approximately 10% of its initial value. This reduction was greater than that achieved with other vegetable fibers such as

wheat bran. It is highly recommended, then, that red beets frequently be included in the diet of individuals wishing to reduce cholesterol levels **(❷,❸).**

• Mild **laxative** due to its fiber content.

• **Aperitif:** Beets increase gastric juice production and tone the stomach.

• **Anticarcinogen:** Doctor Schneider refers to various experiences that took place in Hungary and Germany in which cancerous tumors were reduced or eliminated by administering a daily dose of 250 g of shredded beets or 300-500 ml of juice. These effects were produced even when the juice was boiled and concentrated to make it more tolerable to the stomach, which suggests that whatever the anticarcinogenic substance is, it is heat resistant.

It is very possible that the studies that are in process today concerning the *phytochemicals* in plant-based foods will confirm these experiences and identify the anticarcinogen in red beets.

Figs

Soothe the bronchial passages and invigorate the body

CLASSICAL GREEK athletes, following the recommendation of Galen, ate figs to restore their strength. Today, figs still play a prominent role in the diets of rural Greece, Italy, Spain, and Portugal.

Turkish stevedores, famous for their strength, included figs in their diet back when mechanical aids were not readily available. This is probably the genesis of the popular phrase "He's as strong as a Turk."

In addition to muscular strength, figs provide many other medicinal properties that make them a particularly healthful fruit.

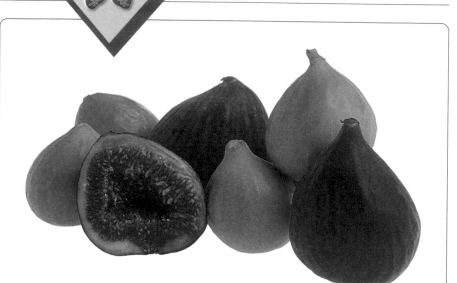

Synonyms: *Common fig, Poor-man's-food;*
French: *Figue;*
Spanish: *Higo, breva;*
German: *Feige.*

Description: *The sweet, fleshy, hollow, pear-shaped, multiple fruit of the fig tree, a deciduous plant ('Ficus carica' L.), having numerous tiny seedlike fruits. It is of the botanical family Moraceae. Certain types of fig trees give two crops a year: the early figs in spring are very tender and juicy. Later figs are harvested in late summer or fall.*

Habitat: *Figs are from hot, semiarid Mediterranean regions. They were introduced to the American continent by Spanish explorers. It acclimated very well to the West Coast of North America. The world's primary producers are Turkey, Greece, Spain, Portugal, and California.*

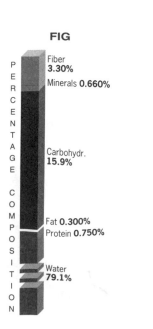

FIG

PERCENTAGE COMPOSITION

Fiber **3.30%**
Minerals **0.660%**
Carbohydr. **15.9%**
Fat **0.300%**
Protein **0.750%**
Water **79.1%**

Preparation and Use

❶ **Fresh:** Figs must be tree-ripened to truly enjoy their sweetness and flavor. If they are harvested green, they will never fully ripen. Fresh figs are only available in the market for a few weeks a year because they are difficult to transport and store.

❷ **Dried:** Dried figs have lost two thirds of their water content, which highly concentrates their sugars, vitamins, and minerals. They are available year-round. Soaking them overnight rehydrates them before eating.

❸ **Boiled in milk** (preferably non-dairy): A half-dozen dried figs cooked in a half-liter of milk is an excellent cough remedy and expectorant, particularly if a few spoonfuls of honey are added.

❹ **Fig cakes:** These are prepared from dried figs, almonds, and aromatic herbs. They provide a great deal of energy and are invigorating to the whole body.

PROPERTIES AND INDICATIONS: *Carbohydrates* are the most significant component in figs, composing 15.9% by weight. Most of these are made up of monosaccharides or simple sugars (glucose and fructose), and a small portion of disaccharides (saccharose). Their proportion of proteins does not reach 1%, and their fat content is only 0.3%.

Figs are quite rich in *vitamins E, B₆, B₁, and B₂*. On the other hand, they are deficient in vitamins A and C. Their more prominent *minerals* are potassium, calcium, magnesium, and iron. *Trace elements* such as zinc, copper, and manganese are present in significant quantities.

Figs are easily digested, and have an emollient (soothing) effect on the bronchial passages and the digestive tract. They are also laxative and diuretic. Fig consumption is particularly indicated in the following cases:

• **Bronchial disorders:** Figs, regardless of how they are prepared, but particularly dried figs that have been rehydrated **❷** or boiled with milk **❸**, have a pectoral action that fights infections.[127] They relieve cough, facilitate expectoration, and soothe the respiratory tract. Their use is recommended in cases of chronic **bronchitis,** as well as acute respiratory infections caused by **colds** or **flu.**

• **Constipation:** Fresh figs **❶** and rehydrated dried figs **❷** are *particularly useful* in cases of slow intestinal peristalsis. They act much in the same way as prunes. They soothe the digestive tract and stimulate peristalsis in the intestine, thus moving the feces.

• **Increase in nutritional need:** Figs in any form are a highly desirable food in cases of anemia or fatigue from physiological or psychological causes because of their invigorating effect.

Pregnant or lactating women, adolescents, and all who are involved in physical (athletes) or psychological (students) activities will find in the fig a highly nutritious, easily digested, and high-energy food.

Applied externally, figs are used for skin disorders as described in the *Encyclopedia of Medicinal Plants* (see *EMP* p. 708) that forms part of the EDUCATION AND HEALTH LIBRARY.

Comparison of the Composition of Fresh and Dried Figs
per 100 g

	fresh	dried
NUTRIENTS WHOSE CONCENTRATION INCREASES WITH DEHYDRATION		
Proteins	0.75	3.05
Fats	0.3	1.17
Carbohydrates	15.9	56.1
Fiber	3.3	9.3
Vitamin B₁	0.06	0.07
Vitamin B₂	0.05	0.09
Vitamin B₆	0.113	0.224
Calcium	35	144
Magnesium	17	59
Iron	0.37	2.23
Calories	74	255
NUTRIENTS WHOSE CONCENTRATION DIMINISHES WITH DEHYDRATION		
Vitamin A	14	13
Vitamin C	2	0.8

FIG Composition
per 100 g of raw edible portion

Energy	74.0 kcal = 310 kj
Protein	0.750 g
Carbohydrates	15.9 g
Fiber	3.30 g
Vitamin A	14.0 µg RE
Vitamin B₁	0.060 mg
Vitamin B₂	0.050 mg
Niacin	0.500 mg NE
Vitamin B₆	0.113 mg
Folate	6.00 µg
Vitamin B₁₂	—
Vitamin C	2.00 mg
Vitamin E	0.890 mg α-TE
Calcium	35.0 mg
Phosphorus	14.0 mg
Magnesium	17.0 mg
Iron	0.370 mg
Potassium	232 mg
Zinc	0.150 mg
Total Fat	0.300 g
Saturated Fat	0.060 g
Cholesterol	—
Sodium	1.00 mg

1% 2% 4% 10% 20% 40% 100%

% Daily Value (based on a 2,000 calorie diet) provided by 100 g of this food

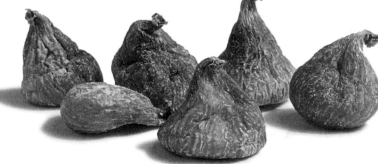

Dried figs concentrate most of their nutrients, with the exception of vitamins E and C, which practically disappear.

Dried figs' medicinal effects on the bronchial passages and the digestive tract are even superior to those of fresh figs.

Carica papaya L.   pH↑

Papaya

Activates the digestive process

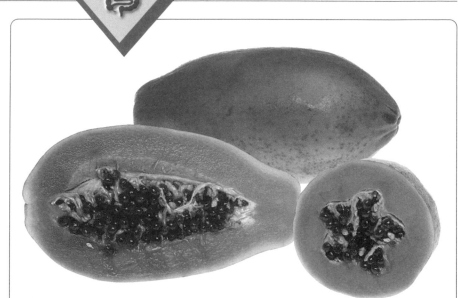

AS THE YEAR 1492 passed, Christopher Columbus found himself in the newly discovered islands of Cuba and Hispaniola (later called Santo Domingo). A whole new fascinating world opened before him and his crew. One of them might have said,

– "Admiral, I've noticed that the natives eat all the meat and fish they want with no ill effect as long as they end each meal with a piece of fruit. It looks like a melon, but it grows on a tree."

Columbus, according to his journal, investigated this custom and found that the natives called the tree *vanti*, which means, "feel well."

Synonyms: *Pawpaw, Melon fruit, Papaw, Melon pawpaw;*
French: *Papaye;*
Spanish: *Papaya, Lechosa, Mamao, melón zapote;*
German: *Papaya.*

Description: *Fruit of 'Carica papaya' L, a fast-growing branchless herb-like tree 3-6 meters in height of the botanical family Caricaceae. The fruit usually weighs 0.5 to 2 kilos, although there are some that reach 6 kilos. The green or yellow rind encloses a delicate yellow or orange pulp. Its center is filled with sour black seeds.*

Habitat: *Papayas are originally from Mexico and the Antilles, where they even grow wild. Their cultivation has spread throughout all tropical areas of the world.*

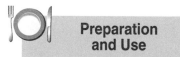

Preparation and Use

❶ **Fresh:** This is the best way to eat papaya. The fruit sold in nontropical countries is normally picked green to facilitate their transport. Consequently, they lose quality and flavor. Papaya makes an excellent breakfast or dessert, although it also goes well in a lettuce salad with lemon juice.

❷ **Other methods of preparation:** The papaya lends itself well to **soft drinks, shakes, and ice cream.** Papaya jam is a popular dessert in the American tropics.

❸ **Canned:** Canned papaya allows it to be enjoyed throughout the world.

PAPAYA
Composition
per 100 g of raw edible portion

Energy	39.0 kcal = 161 kj
Protein	0.610 g
Carbohydrates	8.01 g
Fiber	1.80 g
Vitamin A	175 µg RE
Vitamin B₁	0.027 mg
Vitamin B₂	0.032 mg
Niacin	0.471 mg NE
Vitamin B₆	0.019 mg
Folate	38.0 µg
Vitamin B₁₂	—
Vitamin C	61.8 mg
Vitamin E	1.12 mg α-TE
Calcium	24.0 mg
Phosphorus	5.00 mg
Magnesium	10.0 mg
Iron	0.100 mg
Potassium	257 mg
Zinc	0.070 mg
Total Fat	0.140 g
Saturated Fat	0.043 g
Cholesterol	—
Sodium	3.00 mg

1%   2%   4%   10%   20%   40%   100% 200% 500%

**% Daily Value (based on a 2,000 calorie diet)
provided by 100 g of this food**

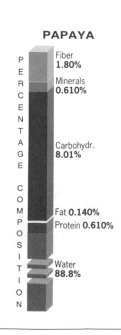

PAPAYA

PERCENTAGE COMPOSITION

Fiber 1.80%
Minerals 0.610%
Carbohydr. 8.01%
Fat 0.140%
Protein 0.610%
Water 88.8%

Today it is known that the papaya contains small amounts of an enzyme that is capable of digesting 200 times its own weight in proteins. It is also known that just because papayas aid the digestion process, they should not be abused as they were by those long-ago Caribbean natives.

PROPERTIES AND INDICATIONS: The papaya in 88.8% water, almost as much as a melon (92%). This is why some call it the "tropical melon." However, the papaya and the melon belong to distinct botanical families with completely different characteristics.

Its content of energy producing nutrients is quite reduced in carbohydrates (8%), proteins (0.61%) and fats (0.14%). Most of its carbohydrates are formed from sugars: saccharose, glucose, and fructose.

Its *vitamin* content, however, is striking: 100 g of pulp provides 103% of the RDA of *vitamin C* and 18% of *vitamin A* for an adult.

The B vitamins are also present in small amounts except for *folates*, which, with 38 mg/100 g, is as much as the mango or the feijoa, the richest fresh fruits in these substances.

Where minerals are concerned, the papaya is *rich* in *potassium* (257 µg /100 g), and significant amounts of calcium, magnesium, phosphorous, and iron. *Pectin* (soluble vegetable fiber) makes 1.8%.

Using sophisticated methods of chemical analysis 106 volatile chemical substances have been identified in papaya pulp that are responsible for its aroma.[128] This figure gives an idea as to just how complex the composition of fruit really is. There are so many substances in plant-based foods whose function is not known, and so many yet to discover!

• *PAPAIN* is a proteolytic enzyme (one that digests proteins), similar to the pepsin in gastric juice. Its primary source is the leaves of the papaya tree or its unripe fruit. Papain is greatly reduced in ripe papayas.

Papaya is *very easy to digest* and contributes to the digestion of other foods. These are its primary therapeutic indications:

• **Stomach disorders:** Papaya is rec-

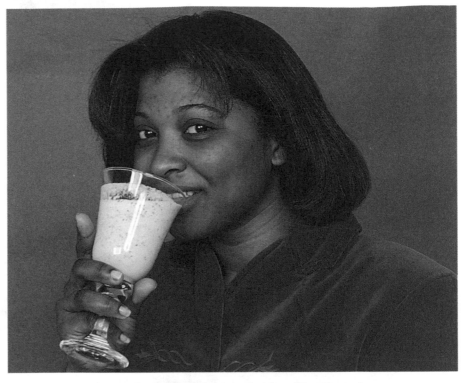

Papaya is considered the perfect breakfast throughout the tropics. Perhaps this is because of its digestibility and vitamin richness. A papaya shake is one of the most pleasant ways of eating this fruit.

ommended in cases of difficult digestion, gastric ptosis (gastric prolapse), gastritis, and anytime digestion is affected by inflammation of the gastric mucosa.

Papaya helps neutralize **excess gastric acid.** Consequently, it is beneficial in cases of **gastroduodenal ulcer, hiatal hernia,** and **pyrosis** (heartburn).

• **Biliary dyspepsia** and chronic **pancreatitis:** Papaya is of value because of its effect on all digestive processes and its very low fat content.

• **Intestinal disorders:** The papaya's emollient and antiseptic effect on the digestive mucosa makes it useful in any type of case of gastroenteritis or colitis: infectious, ulcerous, or spastic (irritable bowel).

Studies carried out in Japan,[129] show that papaya, particularly when it is slightly green, has bacteriostatic properties, impeding the development of many enteropathogens that cause intestinal infections: *Enterobacter cloacae, Escherichia coli, Salmonella typhi, Staphylococcus aureus, Pseudomonas aeruginosa,* and others. Papaya is highly recommended for **infectious diarrhea.**

• **Intestinal parasites:** Papaya sap or *latex,*[130] and to a lesser extent the pulp, have anthelminthic and vermifuge properties against intestinal parasites, particularly tenia (tapeworm).

• **Skin disorders:** Papaya is a part of the suggested diet for those with skin disorders such as eczema, furunculosis, and acne because of its richness in provitamin A.

Cichorium intybus
L. var. foliosum

pH↑

Belgian Endive

Eases digestion for gallbladder patients

The white tenderness of the Belgian endive is the result of depriving it of sunlight. This makes it poorer in vitamins and other nutrients than the green leaves of other varieties of chicory.

Synonyms: *Witloof, French endive, Endive;*
French: *Endive;*
Spanish: *Endivia, achicoria blanca;*
German: *Chicorée.*

Description: *The leaves of the Belgian endive ('Cichorium intybus' L. var. 'foliosum'), a herbaceous plant of the botanical family Compositae. This is a variety of chicory, derived by sprouting its roots in a dark, hot, humid place.*

Habitat: *Endives are cultivated in Belgium, France, The Netherlands, and Germany, as well as in the United States and Canada.*

PERCENTAGE COMPOSITION

Fiber 3.10 %
Minerals 0.470 %
Carbohydr. 0.900 %
Fat 0.100 %
Protein 0.900 %
Water 94.5 %

I T IS SAID that to find the perfect endive, one cannot leave Brussels and must keep the three requirements of the forced cultivation of the vegetable in mind: humidity, heat, and darkness.

The Belgian endive is, in reality, a variety of chicory that is obtained using forced or artificial growing techniques. In the 19th century, Belgian farmers discovered that chicory roots stored in a hot, humid, dark environment produced very tender white sprouts.

PROPERTIES AND INDICATIONS: Belgian endive has a very pleasant texture and flavor. As it is an artificially grown plant, however, it has fewer nutrients and active substances than other chicory varieties, including wild chicory. However, refined Western palates find the white endive more acceptable than other varieties.

Belgian endive is 94.5% water. *Proteins* make up 0.9% of its weight, which is significant since this is a fresh vegetable. Its *carbohydrates,* the most abundant of which is *inulin,* do not reach 1%. Its *fat* content is practically nonexistent (0.1%). Taken together the Belgian endive provides *17 kcal /100 g,* one of the lowest figures of any food.

Preparation and Use

❶ **Raw:** This is the ideal form to eat them. Seasoned with olive oil and lemon, it is a healthful and highly digestible dish.

❷ **Cooked:** either boiled (served with mayonnaise, as asparagus) or baked in the oven as a part of various dishes.

BELGIAN ENDIVE Composition
per 100 g of raw edible portion

Energy	17.0 kcal = 72.0 kj
Protein	0.900 g
Carbohydrates	0.900 g
Fiber	3.10 g
Vitamin A	3.00 µg RE
Vitamin B₁	0.062 mg
Vitamin B₂	0.027 mg
Niacin	0.427 mg NE
Vitamin B₆	0.042 mg
Folate	37.0 µg
Vitamin B₁₂	—
Vitamin C	2.80 mg
Vitamin E	—
Calcium	19.0 mg
Phosphorus	26.0 mg
Magnesium	10.0 mg
Iron	0.240 mg
Potassium	211 mg
Zinc	0.160 mg
Total Fat	0.100 g
Saturated Fat	0.024 g
Cholesterol	—
Sodium	2.00 mg

1% 2% 4% 10% 20% 40% 100%

% Daily Value (based on a 2,000 calorie diet)
provided by 100 g of this food

Belgian endive is a good source of **folic acid** (37 mg/100 g), as well as **vitamin B₁** (thiamin). Vitamins B₂, B₆, and niacin are also present. It contains very little vitamin A or C, as opposed to green-leafed chicory, which are quite rich in these vitamins.

As far as **minerals** are concerned, it contains small amounts of calcium, phosphorous, magnesium, and iron. It is quite rich in potassium and contains the trace elements zinc, copper, and manganese.

Belgian endive contains the same bitter substances that are found in green chicory, but in lower amounts. This is what gives it a slightly bitter taste. These substances act on the liver, increasing bile production (**choleretic** action) and facilitating the drainage of the gallbladder (**cholagogic** action). It also serves as an **aperitif** and a **tonic** for the stomach and digestive functions. This makes Belgian endives useful in the following cases:

• **Gallbladder disorders** due to the presence of calculi (cholelithiasis) or disruption of its proper drainage (biliary dyskinesia). The beneficial action of the bitter substances in the Belgian endive, together with its virtual lack of fat makes it very easy to digest.

• **Diabetes:** Belgian endive is a *perfect* food for diabetics since it contains very few carbohydrates, and those that are present are primarily formed of *fructose* (*inulin* is a polymer of fructose). This simple sugar *requires less* **insulin** to be metabolized, contrary to glucose, which needs more. Consequently, it is very well tolerated by diabetics.

Experiments with laboratory animals[132] show that Belgian endive extracts slow the absorption of glucose in the small intestine. Therefore, diabetics who eat endives along with other foods do not experience sudden increases in blood glucose levels.

• **Obesity:** Belgian endives require a certain amount of chewing and contain very few calories. This makes them very appropriate for weight-loss diets.

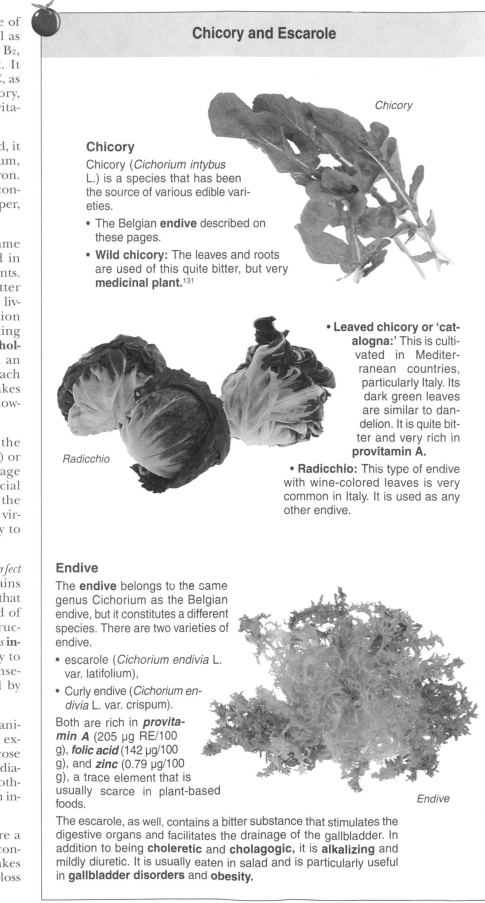

Chicory and Escarole

Chicory

Chicory (*Cichorium intybus* L.) is a species that has been the source of various edible varieties.

• The Belgian **endive** described on these pages.

• **Wild chicory:** The leaves and roots are used of this quite bitter, but very **medicinal plant.**[131]

Chicory

Radicchio

• **Leaved chicory or 'catalogna:'** This is cultivated in Mediterranean countries, particularly Italy. Its dark green leaves are similar to dandelion. It is quite bitter and very rich in **provitamin A.**

• **Radicchio:** This type of endive with wine-colored leaves is very common in Italy. It is used as any other endive.

Endive

The **endive** belongs to the same genus Cichorium as the Belgian endive, but it constitutes a different species. There are two varieties of endive.

• escarole (*Cichorium endivia* L. var. latifolium),

• Curly endive (*Cichorium endivia* L. var. crispum).

Both are rich in **provitamin A** (205 µg RE/100 g), **folic acid** (142 µg/100 g), and **zinc** (0.79 µg/100 g), a trace element that is usually scarce in plant-based foods.

Endive

The escarole, as well, contains a bitter substance that stimulates the digestive organs and facilitates the drainage of the gallbladder. In addition to being **choleretic** and **cholagogic,** it is **alkalizing** and mildly diuretic. It is usually eaten in salad and is particularly useful in **gallbladder disorders** and **obesity.**

Ananas comosus Merr.	pH↑				☿		

Pineapple

The stomach's friend

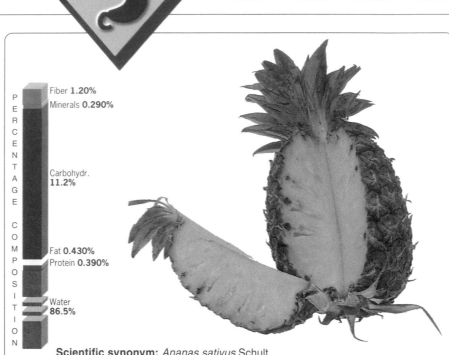

PERCENTAGE COMPOSITION

- Fiber **1.20%**
- Minerals **0.290%**
- Carbohydr. **11.2%**
- Fat **0.430%**
- Protein **0.390%**
- Water **86.5%**

Scientific synonym: *Ananas sativus* Schult.

Synonyms: *Cayenne pineapple, Nana, Ananás;*
French: *Ananas;* **Spanish:** *Ananás, piña [tropical], piña americana;*
German: *Ananas.*

Description: *Compound fruit (formed by the union of the fruits of various blossoms around a central fleshy core) of the pineapple plant ('Ananas comosus' Merr.), a herbaceous plant of the botanical family Bromeliaceae that reaches a height of 50 cm.*

Habitat: *Pineapples are cultivated in tropical regions in America, Asia, and Oceania. Hawaii, Thailand, and Brazil are the main producing regions.*

HISTORY tells that in 1493 the inhabitants of the Antillean island of Guadeloupe offered Christopher Columbus a pineapple, which he took to be a variety of artichoke. He brought it back to Spain, from where it spread to the tropical areas of Asia and Africa. It was first cultivated in Hawaii in the 19th century, which is now one of the primary world producers.

PROPERTIES AND INDICATIONS: Unlike the banana, the pineapple only ripens on the plant. Its content of sugars and active ingredients doubles during its final weeks of ripening. This is why prematurely harvested fruit is acid-tasting and lacks nutritional components. It is best to eat pineapple that has been properly ripened on the plant.

Pineapple that has been properly matured contains approximately 11% carbohydrates, most of which are *sugars*. Their fat and protein contents are negligible.

The prevalent vitamins in pineapple are C, B₁, and B₆. It is also a good source of folates. Among the minerals it contains are manganese (1.65 mg /100 g), followed by copper, potassium, magnesium, and iron.

The pineapple's non-nutritive components are of utmost importance from a dietary and therapeutic standpoint:

✓ *Citric and malic acids:* These are responsible for the pineapple's acidic taste. As is the case with citrus fruits,

PINEAPPLE Composition
per 100 g of raw edible portion

Energy	**49.0 kcal = 207 kj**
Protein	**0.390 g**
Carbohydrates	**11.2 g**
Fiber	**1.20 g**
Vitamin A	**2.00 µg RE**
Vitamin B₁	**0.092 mg**
Vitamin B₂	**0.036 mg**
Niacin	**0.503 mg NE**
Vitamin B₆	**0.087 mg**
Folate	**10.6 µg**
Vitamin B₁₂	**—**
Vitamin C	**15.4 mg**
Vitamin E	**0.100 mg α-TE**
Calcium	**7.00 mg**
Phosphorus	**7.00 mg**
Magnesium	**14.0 mg**
Iron	**0.370 mg**
Potassium	**113 mg**
Zinc	**0.080 mg**
Total Fat	*0.430 g*
Saturated Fat	*0.032 g*
Cholesterol	*—*
Sodium	*1.00 mg*

1% 2% 4% 10% 20% 40% 100%

% Daily Value (based on a 2,000 calorie diet)
provided by 100 g of this food

Preparation and Use

❶ Natural: Pineapple is an ideal dessert, improving digestion. It also is an excellent aperitif, preparing the stomach for a meal.

❷ Juice: Pineapple juice must be drunk slowly because of its acidity.

❸ Canned: Canned pineapple retains most of its vitamins, minerals, and fiber. However, it is poor in the enzyme bromelin, which is easily degraded. As a result, canned pineapple has little effect as a digestive aid.

Pineapple: Choose Well and Gain Greater Benefit

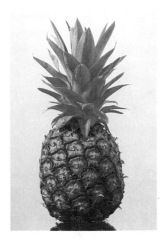

Pineapple only ripens properly on the plant. If it is harvested early to meet the needs of transport, it is very acid and poor in nutrients.

It is important to know how to choose fruit that is ripe. Pineapple is **ripe** when:

1. The **pulp** yields to finger pressure
2. Its **aroma** is intense
3. Its **leaves** are easily removed.

To prepare a pineapple, it must be peeled and cut into 2 cm slices.

Pineapple juice is prepared by placing chunks of pineapple in a blender. The resulting juice should be **drunk** *immediately* to prevent the loss of its properties. It must be drunk *slowly* and well salivated.

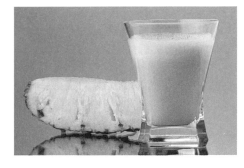

---

they *potentiate* the action of ***vitamin C.*** In spite of its richness in acids, the pineapple acts as an alkalizer from a metabolic standpoint, in other words as an **antacid,** as occurs with the lemon and other citrus fruits.

✓ ***BROMELIN*** (also known as bromelain): This is a protein-digesting enzyme capable of "breaking down" proteins and releasing the amino acids that form them. Because of this, pineapple bromelin has long been used in the food industry as a meat tenderizer.

Bromelin acts in the digestive tract by breaking down *proteins* and *facilitating digestion* in much the same way as the stomach's own pepsin.

The pineapple is a succulent, delicious fruit rich in certain vitamins and minerals. Many consider it a wonderful dessert as an *aid* to the **digestion** of other foods. Others prefer to eat it as an aperitif, eating it before a meal, particularly when the stomach is somehow weakened. Its consumption is specifically indicated for the following conditions:

• **Hypochlorhydria** (scanty gastric juice), which is manifested by slow di-

gestion and a sense of heaviness in the stomach.

• **Gastric ptosis** (prolapsed stomach) caused by the stomach's inability to empty itself (gastric atonia).

In both cases pineapple must be eaten **fresh** (not canned) and **ripe** either before or after a meal.

• **Obesity:** Pineapple or fresh pineapple juice consumed before meals reduces appetite and constitutes a good complement to weight-loss diets. It is also slightly diuretic (facilitates urine production).

• **Sterility:** This tropical fruit is one of the *richest* foods in ***manganese,*** a trace element actively involved in the formation of reproductive cells, both male and female. It is therefore recommended for those suffering from sterility due to insufficient production of germinal cells (sperm in men and ova in women).

• **Stomach cancer:** It has been shown[133] that pineapple is a *powerful* **inhibitor** of the formation of *nitrosamines*. These carcinogenic substances form in the stomach as a chemical reaction between nitrites and certain proteins contained in foods. Nitrosamines are known to be

one of the leading causes of stomach cancer.

Vitamin C alone impedes the formation of nitrosamines, but pineapple (whole or fresh juice) has been shown *much more effective*. Consequently, pineapple is recommended as a preventive for those at high risk for stomach cancer. Those who have suffered from this disease can also benefit from this delicious fruit in preventing recurrence.

Gastroduodenal Ulcer

Pineapple is not recommended during the active phase of a gastroduodenal ulcer since there is usually excess gastric juice present.

Pomegranate

Reduces intestinal inflammation and enriches the blood

THE POMEGRANATE and its color have been the object of great fascination, particularly in Oriental cultures. The Arabs were great admirers and promoters of its cultivation, making it the symbol of the Muslim kingdom of Granada in the southern Iberian Peninsula.

The scarlet blossoms of the pomegranate appear as dazzling flames against the dark green backdrop of the tree's leaves. The tiny beads of fruit, full of precious juice, are brilliant as drops of blood or rubies.

Solomon the wise compared the cheeks of his beloved to the pomegranate three thousand years ago.[126]

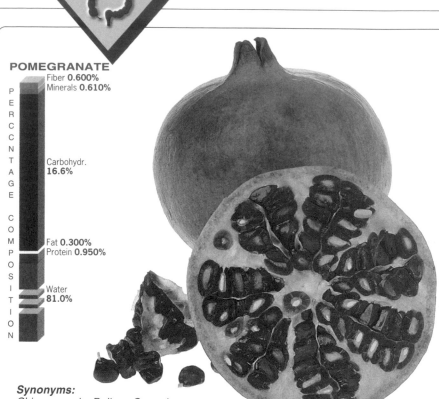

POMEGRANATE

PERCCNTAGE COMPOSITION

Fiber **0.600%**
Minerals **0.610%**
Carbohydr. **16.6%**
Fat **0.300%**
Protein **0.950%**
Water **81.0%**

Synonyms:
Chinese apple, Dalima, Grenade;
French: *Grenade;* **Spanish:** *Granada;*
German: *Granatapfel.*

Description: *Fruit of the pomegranate tree ('Punica granatum' L.), an evergreen belonging to the botanical family Punicaceae that reaches 4 m in height. The fruit is formed of many sacs filled with a very juicy pink or reddish pulp. Each sac contains a seed.*

Habitat: *The pomegranate is originally from the Near East, from where it spread throughout the Mediterranean. It is presently grown in Iran, Turkey, Mediterranean countries and hot regions on the American continent such as Brazil and California.*

POMEGRANATE
Composition
per 100 g of raw edible portion

Energy	**68.0 kcal = 283 kj**
Protein	0.950 g
Carbohydrates	16.6 g
Fiber	0.600 g
Vitamin A	—
Vitamin B₁	0.030 mg
Vitamin B₂	0.030 mg
Niacin	0.300 mg NE
Vitamin B₆	0.105 mg
Folate	6.00 µg
Vitamin B₁₂	—
Vitamin C	6.10 mg
Vitamin E	0.550 mg α-TE
Calcium	3.00 mg
Phosphorus	8.00 mg
Magnesium	3.00 mg
Iron	0.300 mg
Potassium	259 mg
Zinc	0.120 mg
Total Fat	0.300 g
Saturated Fat	0.038 g
Cholesterol	—
Sodium	3.00 mg

1% 2% 4% 10% 20% 40% 100%

% Daily Value (based on a 2,000 calorie diet) provided by 100 g of this food

Preparation and Use

❶ **Natural:** The pomegranate is among the most easily stored fruits after harvest. It ripens well off the tree with little effect on its nutritive properties. Pomegranates stored in a cool, dry place can last up to six months.

If its **anti-parasitic effect** is undesired, the internal membranes that separate the sacs should be removed because of their bitter taste.

❷ **Juice:** Pomegranate juice is very refreshing and flavorful. It is easily extracted using a household juicer.

❸ **Grenadine:** This syrup is made by cooking pomegranate juice with sugar. It may be stored for months. It is used as a beverage, diluted with water, or to flavor fruit salads.

PROPERTIES AND INDICATION: The pomegranate contains an amount of *carbohydrates* that *surpasses* most other fruits: 15.6% (bananas reach 21%). Its *protein* content is close to 1%, which is respectable bearing in mind that this is a fresh fruit. *Fats* are less than 0.3% of its weight.

The pomegranate is quite rich in *vitamins C, E,* and *B₆*, containing, as well, significant amounts of *B₁, B₂,* and *niacin.* It does not contain beta-carotene (provitamin A). The most abundant *minerals* are *potassium, copper,* and *iron.*

Among its non-nutritive components the following are worth noting:

✓ *Tannins,* in small amounts. These are much more prevalent in the **RIND** of the fruit or in the **MEMBRANES** that separate the seed sacs. These tannins have an **astringent** and **anti-inflammatory** effect on the mucosa of the digestive tract.

✓ *Citric acid* and other organic acids which give the pomegranate its pleasant bittersweet taste and a portion of its beneficial effect on the intestine (it contributes to the *restoration* of the intestinal **bacterial flora**).

✓ *Anthocyanins:* These reddish or bluish vegetable pigments belonging to the *flavonoid* group act as **antiseptics** and **anti-inflammatory** substances in the digestive tract and as *potent* **antioxidants** within the cells, *halting* the **aging** process and **cancerous** degeneration. It also has a diuretic effect.

✓ *Pelletierine:* This alkaloid is an effective **vermifuge** (expulses intestinal parasites) that is found primarily in the bark of the **ROOTS** of the tree (see *EMP* [*Encyclopedia of Medicinal Plants*] p. 524). The **RIND** and the **MEMBRANES** also contain this alkaloid, but not the seed sacs.

Together, these components give the pomegranate the following properties: astringent, anti-inflammatory, vermifuge (if the internal membranes are consumed), remineralizer, alkalizer, and depurant.

Its use is particularly indicated in the following cases:

• **Intestinal disorders:** The pomegranate is suitable in cases of **infectious diarrhea** caused by gastroenteritis or colitis because of its astringent

Preparing a Pomegranate

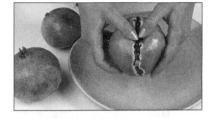
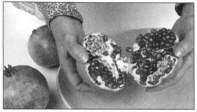

1. Split the fruit in half

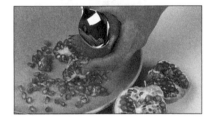
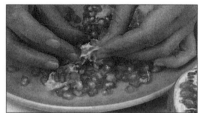

2. Tap the rind with the bottom of a spoon to release the sacs.

3. Remove the membrane fragments that may have come out with the sacs. Add honey, if desired, and eat using a spoon.

The pomegranate is an intestinal astringent and anti-inflammatory. The hard residue that remains in the mouth should not be swallowed since it is indigestible.

and anti-inflammatory action on the digestive tract. It is also beneficial in cases of **flatulence** (excess gas) or intestinal **cramps.** Surprising results have been achieved in chronic cases such as ulcerative colitis or granulomatous colitis (Crohn's disease).

• **Intestinal parasites,** tenia or tapeworm, in particular. If an intense vermifuge effect is required, either a maceration of the **BARK** (see *EMP* p. 524), which is very bitter, or of the inner walls of the pomegranate may be employed.

• **Excess stomach acid:** Because of its astringent action it reduces the production of gastric juice and reduces inflammation in an irritated stomach.

• **Iron deficiency anemia:** The pomegranate contains a significant amount of *copper* (70 µg/100 g), a trace element that *facilitates* the *absorption* of *iron.*

• **Arteriosclerosis:** Because of its rich content of *flavonoids* and *antioxidant* vitamins (C and E), which halt the processes of arterial aging, the pomegranate is recommended in cases of reduced arterial blood flow. It is very beneficial in **heart attack** *prevention* and cardiac health in general.

• **Hypertension:** Because of their *richness* in *potassium* and *virtual absence* of *sodium,* pomegranates are appropriate for those suffering from hypertension. They help avoid excessive numbers of both systolic and diastolic pressure.

• **Metabolic disorders:** Pomegranates are of value in cases of **gout,** excess **uric acid,** and **obesity** because of its **alkalizing** and **depurant** effect.

Cucumis melo L. | pH↑

Melon

A source of living water

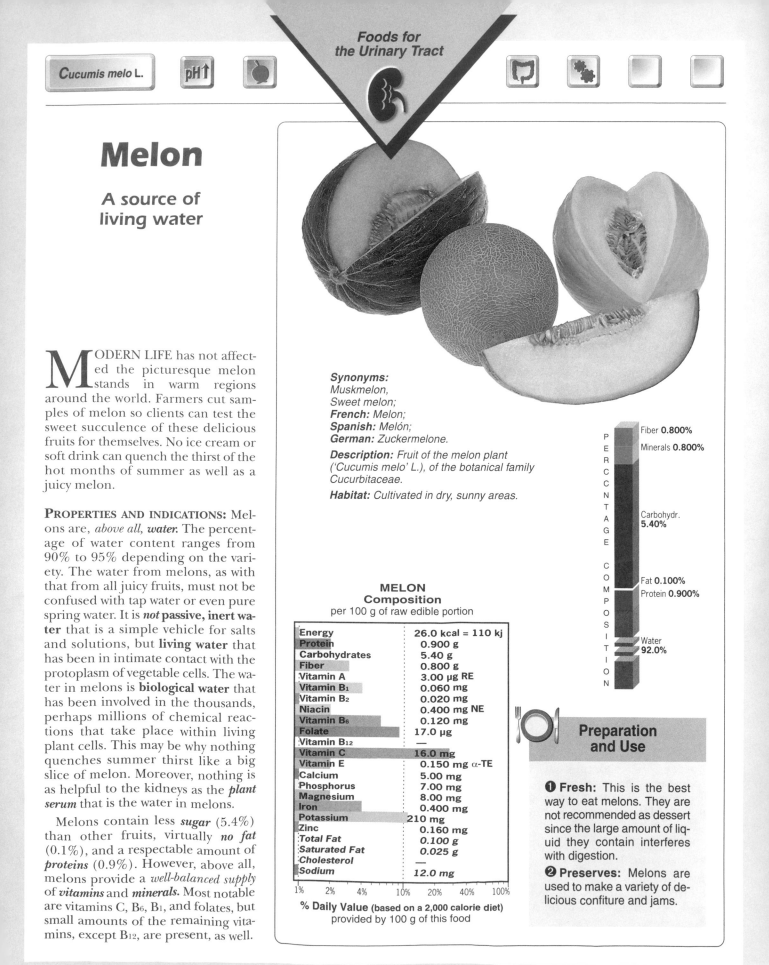

MODERN LIFE has not affected the picturesque melon stands in warm regions around the world. Farmers cut samples of melon so clients can test the sweet succulence of these delicious fruits for themselves. No ice cream or soft drink can quench the thirst of the hot months of summer as well as a juicy melon.

PROPERTIES AND INDICATIONS: Melons are, *above all, water.* The percentage of water content ranges from 90% to 95% depending on the variety. The water from melons, as with that from all juicy fruits, must not be confused with tap water or even pure spring water. It is *not* **passive, inert water** that is a simple vehicle for salts and solutions, but **living water** that has been in intimate contact with the protoplasm of vegetable cells. The water in melons is **biological water** that has been involved in the thousands, perhaps millions of chemical reactions that take place within living plant cells. This may be why nothing quenches summer thirst like a big slice of melon. Moreover, nothing is as helpful to the kidneys as the *plant serum* that is the water in melons.

Melons contain less *sugar* (5.4%) than other fruits, virtually *no fat* (0.1%), and a respectable amount of *proteins* (0.9%). However, above all, melons provide a *well-balanced supply* of *vitamins* and *minerals.* Most notable are vitamins C, B_6, B_1, and folates, but small amounts of the remaining vitamins, except B_{12}, are present, as well.

Synonyms:
Muskmelon,
Sweet melon;
French: *Melon;*
Spanish: *Melón;*
German: *Zuckermelone.*

Description: *Fruit of the melon plant ('Cucumis melo' L.), of the botanical family Cucurtibaceae.*

Habitat: *Cultivated in dry, sunny areas.*

MELON Composition
per 100 g of raw edible portion

Energy	26.0 kcal = 110 kj
Protein	0.900 g
Carbohydrates	5.40 g
Fiber	0.800 g
Vitamin A	3.00 µg RE
Vitamin B_1	0.060 mg
Vitamin B_2	0.020 mg
Niacin	0.400 mg NE
Vitamin B_6	0.120 mg
Folate	17.0 µg
Vitamin B_{12}	—
Vitamin C	16.0 mg
Vitamin E	0.150 mg α-TE
Calcium	5.00 mg
Phosphorus	7.00 mg
Magnesium	8.00 mg
Iron	0.400 mg
Potassium	210 mg
Zinc	0.160 mg
Total Fat	0.100 g
Saturated Fat	0.025 g
Cholesterol	—
Sodium	12.0 mg

1% 2% 4% 10% 20% 40% 100%

% Daily Value (based on a 2,000 calorie diet)
provided by 100 g of this food

PERCENTAGE COMPOSITION

Fiber **0.800%**
Minerals **0.800%**
Carbohydr. **5.40%**
Fat **0.100%**
Protein **0.900%**
Water **92.0%**

Preparation and Use

❶ **Fresh:** This is the best way to eat melons. They are not recommended as dessert since the large amount of liquid they contain interferes with digestion.

❷ **Preserves:** Melons are used to make a variety of delicious confiture and jams.

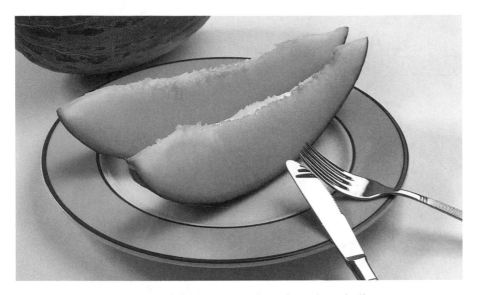

Those who complain that melon gives them indigestion should try eating it before or between meals.

It is better to eat melon before a meal than afterwards as a dessert. Eating it after a meal dilutes gastric juices and puddles the stomach, disturbing digestion.

solubility of the acidic salts that make up uric calculi, and facilitate their dissolution and elimination.

– **Urinary infections** (pyelonephritis, cystitis): Although melons are not urinary antiseptics, their **alkalizing** effect in the urine helps stop the proliferation of the coliform bacilli that cause urinary infections (*Escherichia coli* and others), which require an acidic medium to grow.

• Excess uric acid, manifested by **uratic** (gouty) **arthritis** and **gout.**

• Chronic constipation due to intestinal atony.

• **Dehydration** accompanied by mineral loss, as occurs in diarrhea, excessive perspiration, or fever crises. Although melons are laxative, they may be used without difficulty in case if diarrhea caused by gastroenteritis.

Melons contain all *mineral* nutrients, notably *potassium, iron,* and *magnesium.* One 2.5 kg melon contains the daily need for iron for an adult male (10 mg), and more than half of the magnesium requirement, which is 350 mg.

Melons are hydrating, remineralizing, alkalizing, diuretic, and laxative.

Their most important indications are:

• **Urinary conditions:** Melon consumption enriches the blood with mineral salts and vitamins and facilitates the filtering capacity of the kidneys. After eating melon, the kidneys are better able to effectively remove waste material and toxins produced through metabolic processes. Melons' *"living water"* and their dissolved minerals are major contributors to this. Melons can *benefit* all who wish to improve **renal function** and particularly those suffering from:

– **Early stage kidney failure,** whose primary symptoms are fluid retention and scanty urine output.

– **Kidney stones and granules,** particularly those that are uric in composition. Thanks to their *remarkable* **alkalizing** ability, melons increase the

Cantaloupe

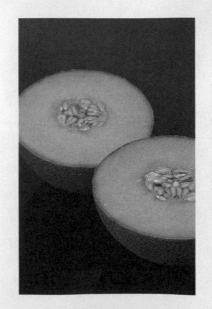

The cantaloupe (*Cucumis melo* L. Var. *cantalupensis*) is a variety of melon appreciated for its characteristic aroma and flavor. Its rind is yellowish green with a type of reticulated relief. The pulp of this melon is orange, and is *very rich* in **beta-carotene** (provitamin A): One hundred grams of cantaloupe provide 332 µg RE, which represents a third of the daily need of this vitamin for an adult male. It contains 90% water, more vitamin C and less iron than common melons. Concentrations of the remaining nutrients are substantially similar.

Cantaloupes are equally effective in treating **urinary conditions,** with the added advantage of their greater beta-carotene content.

__French:__ Melon; __Spanish:__ Melón cantalupo.

Prunus Avium L. | pH↑

Cherry

Satisfies the hunger and purifies the blood

ANYONE WHO has ever had anything to do with cherries knows that when birds start to eat them they are ripe and delicious. A cherry tree in bloom, and later filled with fruit, adds a cheerful note of color to spring. Humans as well as the birds benefit from this bounty.

Cherries have been eaten in Europe since the time of the Greeks and the Romans. Their delicate flavor and the pleasant sensation they leave ex-

Related species: *Prunus cerasus* L. (sour cherry)

French *Cerise;*
Spanish: *Cereza, guinda;*
German: *Kirsche.*

Description: *Fruit of the cherry tree ('Prunus avium' L.), of the botanical family Rosaceae that reaches a height of 20 meters. The fruit is a drupe about 2 cm in diameter whose color varies from light red to deep purple.*

Habitat: *Cherries are native to Central and Southern Europe, where they still may be found wild. Cherry cultivation has spread throughout temperate and cold regions of the world.*

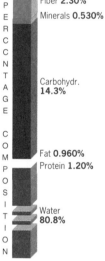

CHERRY

P
E
R
C
C
N
T
A
G
E

C
O
M
P
O
S
I
T
I
O
N

Fiber **2.30%**
Minerals **0.530%**

Carbohydr. **14.3%**

Fat **0.960%**
Protein **1.20%**

Water **80.8%**

CHERRY
Composition
per 100 g of raw edible portion

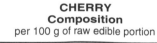

Energy	72.0 kcal = 300 kj
Protein	1.20 g
Carbohydrates	14.3 g
Fiber	2.30 g
Vitamin A	21.0 µg RE
Vitamin B₁	0.050 mg
Vitamin B₂	0.060 mg
Niacin	0.400 mg NE
Vitamin B₆	0.036 mg
Folate	4.20 µg
Vitamin B₁₂	—
Vitamin C	7.00 mg
Vitamin E	0.130 mg α-TE
Calcium	15.0 mg
Phosphorus	19.0 mg
Magnesium	11.0 mg
Iron	0.390 mg
Potassium	224 mg
Zinc	0.060 mg
Total Fat	0.960 g
Saturated Fat	0.216 g
Cholesterol	—
Sodium	2.00 mg

1%   2%   4%   10%   20%   40%   100%

% Daily Value (based on a 2,000 calorie diet) provided by 100 g of this food

Preparation and Use

❶ **Fresh:** Cherries must be eaten one by one, chewing them well.

❷ **Cherry treatment:** This is done by eating one-half kg of ripe cherries as the only food three or four times a day for two or three days. Those with **delicate stomachs** may **boil** them before eating. For a *stronger effect,* one may drink several cups of a tea made by **boiling** 50 g of **cherry stems** in a liter of water for 5 minutes.

❸ **Culinary recipes:** Cherries fit perfectly into a variety of fruit pies, jams, and compotes.

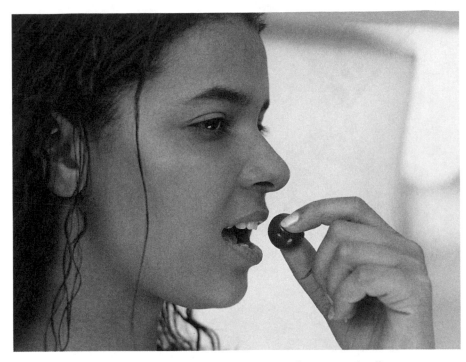

A treatment with cherries one or two days a week allows weight loss while purifying the body and cleansing the blood. The slowness with which cherries must be eaten partially explains their satiating effect.

plain why they are popular on the five continents, although the cherry tree does not do well in tropical regions.

PROPERTIES AND INDICATIONS: Traditionally cherries have been considered a sweet, pleasant fruit, but one of little nutritional or dietetic importance.

However, it is now known that, while none of its nutrients is particularly outstanding, it contains *all* of them in *small amounts* (except for vitamin B12). Of its 14% *sugars,* the most important is fructose, which makes cherries appropriate for diabetics. *Fats* and *proteins* represent about 1% each.

Cherries contain small amounts of vitamins A, B, C, and E, as well as all minerals and trace elements: calcium, phosphorus, magnesium, iron, sodium, *potassium* (the most abundant), zinc, copper, and manganese.

However, cherries also contain small amounts of non-nutritive components:

✓ *Organic acids:* Malic, succinic, and citric, which act as **stimulants** to the digestive glands and as blood **purifiers.** Light red cherries are richer in these acids than darker varieties. Sour cherries (*Prunus cerasus* L.) contain much more.

✓ *Soluble vegetable fiber,* which is formed primarily of pectin. One hundred grams of cherries provide 10% of RDA (Recommended Daily Allowance) of vegetable fiber. This explains their gentle **laxative** and **hypolipedemic** (cholesterol lowering) effects.

✓ *Flavonoids* that give them **diuretic, antioxidant,** and **anticarcinogenic** properties. Among these flavonoids, *elagic acid* is the most noteworthy. According to current research, this substance has the capacity to neutralize carcinogenic substances, preventing healthy cells from becoming cancerous.

✓ *Salicylic acid,* the natural precursor to aspirin, acts as an **anti-inflammatory** and **antirheumatic.** It is present in very small amounts, around 2 mg per kg of cherries, but sufficient to have an effect.

Cherries are a pleasant, easy-to-eat fruit. They are particularly beneficial in the following cases:

• **Obesity:** The fact that cherries must be eaten one by one makes them effective in cases of obesity. Eating 360 calories of pastry only requires a few bites. On the other hand, eating the same amount of calories in the form of cherries means one-half kilo (about one pound). This may take 15 minutes and result in a much greater feeling of satiety than after eating the sweet, eliminating the desire to continue eating.

Cherries' **diuretic** and **depurant** (purifying) effect, coupled with their virtual lack of *sodium* and *fats, potentiate* their **weight loss effect.**

• **Diabetes:** Diabetics tolerate controlled amounts of cherries very well since *half* of their *sugars* are *fructose.* As in the case of all fruit treatments, that associated with cherries [❷] is not recommended for diabetics except under professional supervision.

• **Depurant (purifying) treatments** [❷]: According to Dr. *Valnet,* a distinguished French phytotherapist, one or two days of treatment with cherries represents an excellent depurant (purifier) for the body in general, which facilitates the elimination of wastes and toxins.

• **Chronic disorders:** **Ample** use of cherries, particularly as a **weekly treatment** [❷], is recommended for all types of chronic conditions such as arthritis, gout, chronic rheumatism, arteriosclerosis, chronic constipation, autointoxication due to improper diet, chronic hepatopathy, cardiac failure, convalescence from infectious disease, and cancer.

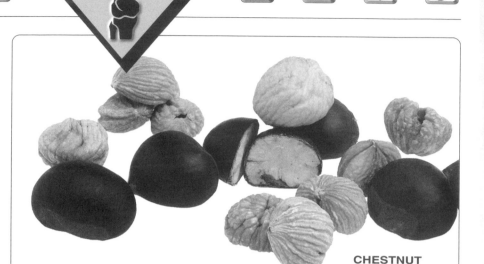

Castanea sativa Mill.

Chestnut

Invigorates the muscles

T HE GERMAN physician and nutritionist W. Heupke, considered one of the founders of the modern German school of nutrition, called chestnuts "the small loaves of bread that nature provides."[124]

In times of famine or war when bread was scarce, many Europeans survived on chestnuts, using its flour to make a bread substitute. In fact, the chestnut, which is botanically a nut or seed, has a composition much more similar to grains than to other nuts.

French: *Châtaigne;*
Spanish: *Castaña;*
German: *Kastanie.*

Description: *Seed of the fruit of the chestnut tree ('Castanea sativa' Mill.), a robust tree of the botanical family Fagaceae.*

Habitat: *The chestnut is from the mountainous regions of Turkey, from where it spread through Southern and Central Europe. It is also cultivated in the South and Eastern United States, China, and Japan.*

CHESTNUT

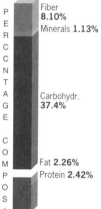

PERCENTAGE COMPOSITION

- Fiber **8.10%**
- Minerals **1.13%**
- Carbohydr. **37.4%**
- Fat **2.26%**
- Protein **2.42%**
- Water **48.7%**

CHESTNUT
Composition
per 100 g of raw edible portion

Energy	213 kcal = 890 kj
Protein	2.42 g
Carbohydrates	37.4 g
Fiber	8.10 g
Vitamin A	3.00 µg RE
Vitamin B1	0.238 mg
Vitamin B2	0.168 mg
Niacin	1.63 mg NE
Vitamin B6	0.376 mg
Folate	62.0 µg
Vitamin B12	—
Vitamin C	43.0 mg
Vitamin E	—
Calcium	27.0 mg
Phosphorus	93.0 mg
Magnesium	32.0 mg
Iron	1.01 mg
Potassium	518 mg
Zinc	0.520 mg
Total Fat	2.26 g
Saturated Fat	0.425 g
Cholesterol	—
Sodium	3.00 mg

1%   2%   4%   10%   20%   40%   100%

% de la CDR (cantidad diaria recomendada)
cubierta por 100 g de este alimento

Preparation and Use

❶ **Raw:** Chestnuts should only be eaten raw when they are *very tender,* and even then they must be very well chewed to begin digestion in the mouth.

❷ **Cooked:** Once shelled, they are boiled for 20-30 min. Aromatic herbs such as cumin, fennel, or thyme may be added to the water.

❸ **Roasted** either in the oven or over coals. They may be roasted with the shell, which must be cut to relieve pressure. Roasted chestnuts are delicious.

❹ **Chestnut puree:** After boiling, the chestnuts are mashed to a consistent paste. Brown sugar or honey may be added. The paste may also be mixed with milk.

❺ **'Marron glacé'** is a classic exquisite French sweet made from the best quality chestnuts and egg white.

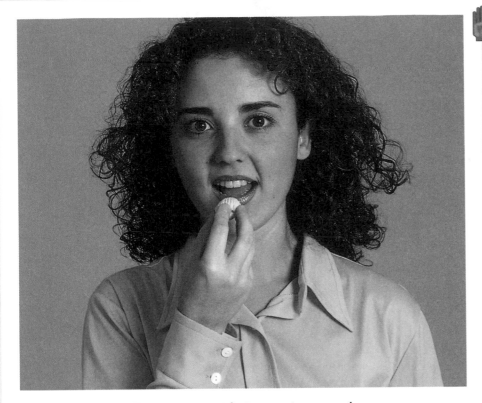

Chestnuts are not just a sweet or a snack, but a very nutritious and invigorating food.

Chew them Well

The chestnut's **carbohydrates, starch,** and **saccharose** must be treated with digestive enzymes to be converted into **simple sugars** that can pass to the bloodstream. If chestnuts are not well chewed, mixing them well with saliva, undigested fragments can reach the large intestine causing flatulence.

Because of this, chestnuts must be chewed thoroughly and well mixed with saliva before swallowing. Boiling, roasting, or particularly pureeing makes them **more digestible.**

The **obese** and **diabetics** must exercise **caution** when eating chestnuts because of this nut's carbohydrate richness.

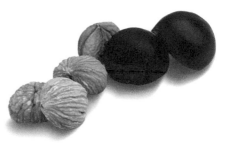

PROPERTIES AND INDICATIONS: The chestnut is one of nature's *richest carbohydrate* sources (37.4%), *comparable only* to **legumes** and **grains.** These carbohydrates are formed primarily of *starch* (85%), and *saccharose* (15%). There is virtually no glucose or fructose.

Chestnuts also contain proteins (2.42%) and fats (2.26%), most of which are mono and polyunsaturated. They provide 213 kcal/100 g, an amount that is considerably higher than the potato (79 kcal/100 g), although less than wheat flour (364 kcal /100 g) or walnuts (642 kcal/100 g).

Even though they contain no vitamin E and little vitamin A, they are quite rich in vitamin C and, above all, in B complex vitamins: B_1, B_2, B_6, and niacin. This *B vitamin* concentration is *similar* to that of **whole wheat** (including the germ).

The chestnut's mineral content is noteworthy for its *richness* in *potassium* (518 mg/100 g) and its *low sodium content* (3 mg/100 g), which makes it *very beneficial* for those with **hypertension** or **cardiovascular disorders.** It also contains a significant amount of iron (1 mg/100 g), as well as magnesium, calcium, phosphorus, and the trace elements zinc, copper, and manganese.

Chestnuts act as a muscle tonic, **alkalizer,** astringent, and galactagogue (promotes milk flow).

Chestnuts are indicated in the following cases:

• **Physical fatigue** due to intense muscular exercise (athletes, manual laborers) or malnutrition. They have a tonic effect on the muscles, providing a sensation of energy and well-being.

• **Growth periods:** Chestnuts are a good source of the calories, vitamins, and minerals needed for musculoskeletal development of adolescents.

• **Arteriosclerosis** and cardiovascular conditions: Chestnuts provide energy but *very little fat and sodium.* Their *high potassium content* helps prevent hypertension.

• **Diarrhea:** Chestnut puree [❹], in particular, is an excellent food in cases of diarrhea because of its mild astringent and regulating effects.

• **Kidney failure:** When the kidney does not perform properly, there is, among other things, an accumulation of acidic substances in the blood. Among these **are uric acid** and **urea.** Chestnuts are a recommended food for those suffering from kidney failure because their **alkalizing** effect partially compensates for excess acid in the blood. They also contain *little protein* in relation to the energy they provide, which is beneficial in cases of kidney failure.

• **Lactating mothers:** Chestnuts are galactagogues (they promote milk flow). They also provide a great deal of nutrition to the lactating mother.

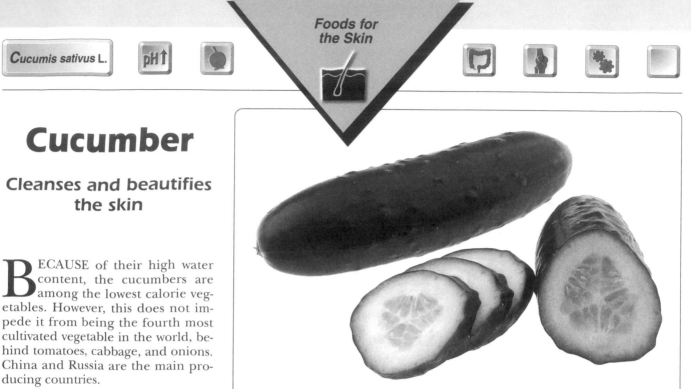

Cucumber

Cleanses and beautifies the skin

BECAUSE of their high water content, the cucumbers are among the lowest calorie vegetables. However, this does not impede it from being the fourth most cultivated vegetable in the world, behind tomatoes, cabbage, and onions. China and Russia are the main producing countries.

The cucumber is native to the south of Asia, although it spread rapidly throughout the ancient world. The Egyptians, the Greeks, and the Romans knew and enjoyed them.

French: *Concombre;* **Spanish:** *Pepino;* **German:** *Gurke.*

Description: *Fruit of the 'Cucumis sativus' L., a herbaceous vine of the botanical family Cucurbitaceae that reaches approximately one meter in height. Cucumbers are eaten unripe since ripe specimens lose their crispness and become spongy and yellow. They measure from 15 to 25 cm in length and about 5 cm in diameter.*

Habitat: *Cucumbers are grown throughout the world both in fresh air and in greenhouses.*

Preparation and Use

❶ **Raw:** Cucumbers are usually eaten this way. Since they are harvested unripe, they must be well chewed to prevent indigestion. They may be eaten in salad with oil and lemon or blended with tomato and other vegetables to make gazpacho. They should be *peeled* to avoid pesticide residue if they have not been organically grown.

❷ **Cooked:** They may be baked with cheese, used in soups, or cooked with other vegetables.

❸ **Pickled:** A particular type of smaller cucumber is prepared in salt and vinegar to preserve them. Because of these two products, pickles are rather unhealthful.

CUCUMBER
Composition
per 100 g of raw edible portion

Energy	13.0 kcal = 53.0 kj
Protein	0.690 g
Carbohydrates	1.96 g
Fiber	0.800 g
Vitamin A	21.0 µg RE
Vitamin B₁	0.024 mg
Vitamin B₂	0.022 mg
Niacin	0.304 mg NE
Vitamin B₆	0.042 mg
Folate	13.0 µg
Vitamin B₁₂	—
Vitamin C	5.30 mg
Vitamin E	0.079 mg α-TE
Calcium	14.0 mg
Phosphorus	20.0 mg
Magnesium	11.0 mg
Iron	0.260 mg
Potassium	144 mg
Zinc	0.200 mg
Total Fat	0.130 g
Saturated Fat	0.034 g
Cholesterol	—
Sodium	2.00 mg

1% 2% 4% 10% 20% 40% 100%

% Daily Value (based on a 2,000 calorie diet) provided by 100 g of this food

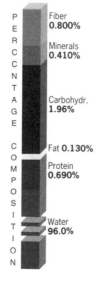

CUCUMBER

PERCENTAGE COMPOSITION

Fiber 0.800%
Minerals 0.410%
Carbohydr. 1.96%
Fat 0.130%
Protein 0.690%
Water 96.0%

Eating a cucumber is like drinking a glass of water. Bearing in mind that 96% of its weight is water, a 250-g cucumber contains 240 g of water. However, this does not mean that it is of little nutritional value! Those 10 grams of solid material in a 250-g cucumber are of *great* **biological** *value* and **healing power.**

PROPERTIES AND INDICATIONS: Cucumbers are among the *most water-rich* foods, and as a result only contain 13 kcal/ 100 g. Their protein (0.69%), carbohydrate (1.96%), and fat (0.13%) content is very low. They also contain small amounts of provitamin A, and vitamins B, C, and E.

Their high *dietary and therapeutic value* resides in their **minerals,** which are **highly alkaline.** They contain potassium, calcium, phosphorus, magnesium, and iron, as well as various trace elements, most notably **sulfur.**

Cucumbers have the following medicinal properties:

– **Alkalizer:** They neutralize excess acidic waste produced in the body as a consequence of the consumption of animal-based foods.
– **Depurant:** They facilitate the elimination of waste substances from the bloodstream through either the urine or the skin.

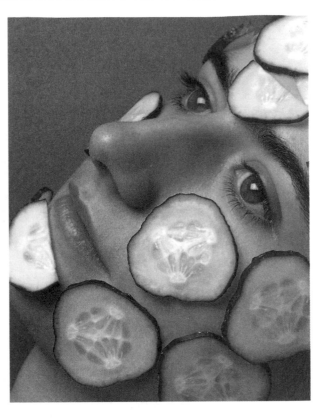

The health and beauty of the skin depend more of the purity of the blood than on the topical application of cosmetic products. True beauty comes from the inside.

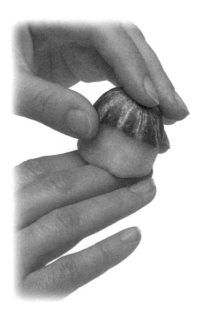

– **Diuretic:** They increase urine output.
– **Laxative:** Given their high water content (96%) and soluble fiber content (0.8%), they facilitate the movement of the feces through the intestine.

These are cucumbers' primary applications:

• **Skin conditions:** Cucumbers hydrate the skin and provide the *sulfur* needed for healthy skin cells, **nails,** and **hair.** At the same time, they **"cleanse" the bloodstream** of toxic wastes. They are recommended for all who are suffering from eczema, dermatosis, and psoriasis. Applied locally directly on the skin, cucumbers are an effective **beauty** treatment.

The best results are obtained by combining cucumbers' internal properties and their external effect on the skin. This is done by:

– Rubbing it directly on the skin.
– Preparing thin slices and placing them on affected skin areas.

• **Constipation** due to intestinal atony.

• **Excess uric acid** and a diet rich in animal-based foods, since it facilitates the elimination of uric acid and other waste substances.

• **Obesity,** because they contain very few calories and produce a certain feeling of satiety.

• **Diabetes,** because of their low carbohydrate content while providing a certain amount of vitamins and minerals.

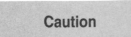

Caution

*Cucumbers are **somewhat indigestible** and may not be well tolerated by those suffering from **dyspepsia** or that have a **frail stomach**. The fact that they are usually eaten green contributes to this problem.*

*To improve tolerance they should be **well chewed**, and specimens that are too green and bitter should be **avoided**. They should **always** be peeled.*

Tangerine

Difficult to eat just one

PEELING and eating tangerines is so simple that it is a favorite fruit of children. Its pleasant sweetness, and low acidity combined with its tender pulp make this citrus one of the most popular in the world.

Tangerines have been raised in Southern Europe, North Africa, and North America since the nineteenth century when they arrived from China. This is the latest species of citrus to arrive in the West from China (oranges were introduced in Europe in the 16th century).

PROPERTIES AND INDICATIONS: The tangerine's composition is *very similar* to that of the **orange** (see Vol. 2, p. 360), although vitamin C, minerals, organic acids, and most other *nutrients* are found in *lower proportions.*

The tangerine's properties are also the *same* as the **orange** although less intense. Consequently, tangerines fight infections, make the blood more fluid, are hypotensive, laxative, antiallergenic, remineralizing, depurant (purifying), and anticarcinogenic. Because they are so easy to eat and digest, they are *particularly* beneficial for **children** and the **elderly.**

Tangerines have two notable applications:

• **Childhood fevers,** because of their ability to fight infection, reinvigorate the body, and replace lost minerals. They are highly recommended in cases of **colds, flu,** and **throat infections.**

• **Hypertension:** Tangerine treatment **[❷]** provides excellent results in cases of hypertension and arteriosclerosis.

PERCCNTAGE COMPOSITION

Fiber **2.30%**

Minerals **0.390%**

Carbohydr. **8.89%**

Fat **0.190%**
Protein **0.630%**

Water **87.6%**

Description: *Fruit of the tangerine tree ('Citrus reticulata' Blanco), a tree of the botanical family Rutaceae that is very similar to the orange tree, although somewhat smaller and more fragile. The two best-known varieties are the satsuma, which is light orange or greenish in color, and the clementine, which is smaller, sweeter, and deep orange in color.*

Habitat: *Native to China, the tangerine has adapted very well to the Mediterranean region and temperate areas of the Americas.*

TANGERINE Composition
per 100 g of raw edible portion

Energy	**44.0 kcal = 184 kj**
Protein	**0.630 g**
Carbohydrates	**8.89 g**
Fiber	**2.30 g**
Vitamin A	**92.0 µg RE**
Vitamin B₁	**0.105 mg**
Vitamin B₂	**0.022 mg**
Niacin	**0.260 mg NE**
Vitamin B₆	**0.067 mg**
Folate	**20.4 µg**
Vitamin B₁₂	—
Vitamin C	**30.8 mg**
Vitamin E	**0.240 mg α-TE**
Calcium	**14.0 mg**
Phosphorus	**10.0 mg**
Magnesium	**12.0 mg**
Iron	**0.100 mg**
Potassium	**157 mg**
Zinc	**0.240 mg**
Total Fat	**0.190 g**
Saturated Fat	**0.022 g**
Cholesterol	—
Sodium	**1.00 mg**

1%   2%   4%   10%   20%   40%   100%

% Daily Value (based on a 2,000 calorie diet)
provided by 100 g of this food

Preparation and Use

❶ Fresh: Peeling and eating tangerines while enjoying their aroma is a true delight. To gain the full benefit of their therapeutic value, one should eat 6 to 8 a day.

❷ Tangerine treatment: As is the case with an orange treatment, this is done by eating 1.5 to 2 kilos (about 3 to 4 pounts) of tangerines as the only food for one or two days a week for a month. Additional liquids should be unnecessary with this amount of fruit since this treatment is usually done in fall or winter.

Citrus
To Eat and Drink

All sour or citrus fruits share in common their sweet and sour flavor, their refreshing juices, and the fact that they are available for most of the year.

The dietetic and therapeutic properties of all citrus fruits are very similar, which is due to a balanced combination of vitamin C, minerals, and phytochemicals.

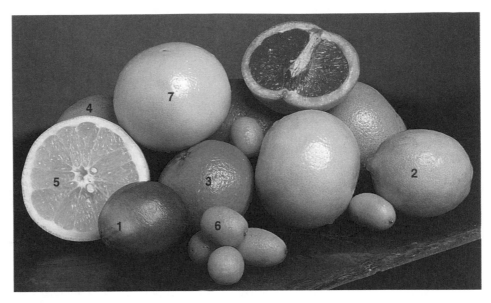

Lime [1]

Citrus aurantiifolia (Christm.-Panz.) Sw. = *Limonia aurantiifolia* Christm.-Panz.

French: *Lime, limette;* ***Spanish:*** *Lima;* ***German:*** *Süße Zitrone.*

The lime is similar in color, size, and shape to the lemon, but its flavor is less sour and much sweeter. It is grown primarily in Central America, Florida, and California.

Its ***vitamin C*** and ***B*** content is *somewhat inferior.* It is used for beverages because of its pleasant aroma.

Lemon [2]

Citrus limon (L.) Burm.

Possibly the citrus with the *most scientifically proved* **medicinal applications.**

Tangerine [3]

Citrus reticulata Blanco

This is the sweetest and mildest-flavored citrus.

Bitter Orange [4]

Citrus aurantium L. = *Citrus vulgaris* Risso.

Synonyms: *Seville orange;* ***French:*** *Orange amère;* ***Spanish:*** *Naranja amarga, naranja agria;* ***German:*** *Bittere Orange.*

These are not edible raw because of their strong flavor. They are only used in confectionery and jellies.

The bitter orange is the one *most used* for **phytotherapeutic** purposes since its **leaves, blossoms,** and **peel** contain high concentrations of *essences* and other *active substances.*

Orange [5]

Citrus sinensis Osbeck.

This is the most widely cultivated and valued citrus. It is described in detail on these pages.

Kumquat [6]

Fortunella margarita (Lour.) Sw.

Related species: *Fortunella japonica [Thunb.] Sw.* (round kumquat)

Synonyms: *Oval kumquat;* ***Spanish:*** *Naranjita china, kumquat [oval].*

These are grown especially in Indonesia, Australia, and Florida. Their size varies between 2 and 3 cm in diameter.

Kumquats are eaten with the skin, which is soft and slightly acid. It is an aromatic and pleasant fruit.

Grapefruit (Vol. 2, p. 93) [7]

Citrus paradisi MacFad. = *Citrus maxima* (Burm.) Merr. = *Citrus decumanus* L.

Grapefruits are effective against **arteriosclerosis.** They are used in **weight loss diets** because of their **detoxifying** properties.

■ ■ ■

Calamondin

Citrus mitis Blanco

Spanish: *Calamondín, lima filipina.*

This citrus is grown in tropical countries. It is orange in color and measures about 2.5 cm in diameter. It is very juicy with a slightly bitter taste. It is used to make beverages and jellies.

Citron

Citrus medica L.

Spanish: *Cidra, toronja;* ***Al.:*** *Zitrone.*

This was the first citrus introduced in Europe, brought from Asia by Alexander the Great in 300 B.C.

Its fruits are large, weighing as much as two kilos. The peel is typically yellow, very thick and wrinkled.

Although it contains *less* **vitamin C** than other citrus, its *calcium content is higher.* Its culinary use is very limited, primarily to provide aroma to pastries such as the famous plum cake.

BIBLIOGRAPHY

Journal references

Author → Article title

SABATÉ, J. ET AL. Effects of walnuts on serum lipid levels and blood pressure in normal men. *N. Engl. J. Med.,* **328:** 603-607 (1993).

Publication date — Publication name — Volume — Beginning and ending pages of article

Book references

Author → Book title

ENSMINGER, A.H. ET AL. *The Concise Encyclopedia of Foods and Nutrition.* Boca Raton, (Florida), CRC Press, 1995.

City of publication — Publisher — Publication date

1. Genesis 1: 29.
2. Genesis 3: 18.
3. NOBMANN, E.D.; BYERS, T.; LANIER, A.P. ET AL. The diet of Alaska Native adults: 1987-1988 [see comments]. *Am. J. Clin. Nutr.,* **55:** 1024-1032 (1992).
4. HEBER, D. The stinking rose: organosulfur compounds and cancer. *Am. J. Clin. Nutr.,* **66:** 425-426 (1997).
5. BERGMAN, J. Diet, Health and Evolution. *Creation Research Society Quarterly,* **34:** 209-217 (1998).
6. MARTINS, Y.; PELCHAT, M.L.; PLINER, P. "Try it; it´s good and it's good for you" effects of taste and nutrition information on willingness to try novel foods. *Appetite,* **28:** 89-102 (1997).
7. REDDY, N.S.; HOTWANI, M.S. In vitro availability of iron from selected nuts and oilseeds. *Plant Foods Hum. Nutr.,* **43:** 247-250 (1993).
8. ABBEY, M. ET AL. Partial replacement of saturated fatty acids with almonds or walnuts lowers total plasma cholesterol and low-density-lipoprotein cholesterol. *Am. J. Clin. Nutr.,* **59:** 995-999 (1994).
9. SABATE, J. ET AL. Effects of walnuts on serum lipid levels and blood pressure in normal men. *N. Engl. J. Med.,* **328:** 603-607 (1993).
10. SPILLER, G.A. ET AL. Effect of a diet high in monounsaturated fat from almonds on plasma cholesterol and lipoproteins. *J. Am. Coll. Nutr.,* **11:** 126-130 (1992).
11. GARG, A. ET AL. Effects of varying carbohydrate content of diet in patients with non-insulin-dependent diabetes mellitus. *JAMA,* **271:** 1421-1428 (1994).
12. KASHTAN, H. ET AL. Wheat-bran and oat-bran supplements´ effects on blood lipids and lipoproteins. *Am. J. Clin. Nutr.,* **55:** 976-980 (1992).
13. SLAVIN, J.L. Epidemiological evidence for the impact of whole grains on health. *Crit. Rev. Food Sci. Nutr.,* **34:** 427-434 (1994).
14. RASANEN, L. Allergy to ingested cereals in atopic children. *Allergy,* **49:** 871-876 (1994).
15. SANDBERG, A.S. The effect of food processing on phytate hydrolysis and availability of iron and zinc. *Adv. Exp. Med. Biol.,* **289:** 499-508 (1991).
16. TORRE, M.; RODRIGUEZ, A.R.; SAURA-CALIXTO, F. Effects of dietary fiber and phytic acid on mineral availability. *Crit. Rev. Food Sci. Nutr.,* **30:** 1-22 (1991).
17. LAMPE, J.W. ET AL. Effects of cereal and vegetable fiber feeding on potential risk factors for colon cancer. Cancer Epidemiol. *Biomarkers Prev.,* **1:** 207-211 (1992).
18. JACOBS, D.R. JR; SLAVIN, J.; MARQUART, L. Whole grain intake and cancer: a review of the literature. *Nutr. Cancer,* **24:** 221-229 (1995).
19. SLAVIN, J.L. Whole grains and health: separating the wheat from the chaff. *Nutr. Today,* **29:** 6-11 (1994).
20. THOMPSON, L.U. Antioxidants and hormone-mediated health benefits of whole grains. *Crit. Rev. Food Sci. Nutr.,* **34:** 473-497 (1994).
21. SALMERON, J. ET AL. Dietary fiber, glycemic load, and risk of NIDDM in men. *Diabetes Care,* **20:** 545-550 (1997).
22. NIELSEN, S.S.; LIENER, I.E. Effect of germination on trypsin inhibitor and hemoagglutinating activities in Phaseolus vulgaris. *J. Food Sci.,* **53:** 298-301 (1988).
23. KHADER, V. Nutritional studies on fermented, germinated and baked soybean preparations. *J. Plant Foods* **5:** 31-37 (1983).
24. BATRA, V. Effects of cooking and germination on hemagglutinin activity in lentil. *Ind. J. Nutr. Diet.,* **24:** 15-19 (1987).
25. SANDBERG, A.S. The effect of food processing on phytate hydrolysis and availability of iron and zinc. *Adv. Exp. Med. Biol.,* **289:** 499-508 (1991).
26. STORY, J.A. ET AL. Interactions of alfalfa plant and sprout saponins with cholesterol in vitro and in cholesterol-fed rats. *Am. J. Clin. Nutr.,* **39:** 917-929 (1984).
27. SIDHU, G.S.; OAKENFULL, D.G. A mechanism for the hypocholesterolaemic activity of saponins. *Br. J. Nutr.,* **55:** 643-649 (1986).
28. RAO, A.V.; SUNG, M.K. Saponins as anticarcinogens. *J. Nutr.,* **125** (3 Suppl): 717S-724S (1995).
29. MAHON, B.E. ET AL. An international outbreak of Salmonella infections caused by alfalfa sprouts grown from contaminated seeds. *J. Infect. Dis.,* **175:** 876-882 (1997).
30. BEUCHAT, L.R. Comparison of chemical treatments to kill Salmonella on alfalfa seeds destined for sprout production. *Int. J. Food Microbiol.,* **34:** 329-333 (1997).
31. JAQUETTE, C.B.; BEUCHAT, L.R.; MAHON, B.E. Efficacy of chlorine and heat treatment in killing Salmonella stanley inoculated onto alfalfa seeds and growth and survival of the pathogen during sprouting and storage. *Appl. Environ. Microbiol.,* **62:** 2212-2215 (1996).
32. HEANEY, R. ET AL. Absorability of calcium from Brassica vegetables: broccoli, bok choy, and kale. *J. Food Sci.,* **58:** 1379-1380 (1993).
33. OOSTHUIZEN, W. ET AL. Both fish oil and olive oil lowered plasma fibrinogen in women with high baseline fibrinogen levels. *Thromb. Haemost.,* **72:** 557-562 (1994).
34. LICHTENSTEIN, A.H. Effects of canola, corn, and olive oils on fasting and postprandial plasma lipoproteins in humans as part of a National Cholesterol Education Program Step 2 diet. *Arterioscler. Thromb.,* **13:** 1533-1542 (1993).
35. REAVEN, P. ET AL. Effect of antioxidants alone and in combination with monounsaturated fatty acid-enriched diets on lipoprotein oxidation. *Arteriosclerosis, Thrombosis and Vascular Biology,* **16:** 1465-1472 (1996).
36. BONANOME, A. ET AL. Effect of dietary monounsaturated and polyunsaturated fatty acids on the susceptibility of plasma low density lipoproteins to oxidative modification. *Arterioscler. Thromb.,* **12:** 529-533 (1992).
37. REAVEN, P.D.; GRASSE, B.J.; TRIBBLE, D.L. Effects of linoleate-enriched and oleate-enriched diets in combination with alpha-tocopherol on the susceptibility of LDL and LDL subfractions to oxidative modification in humans. *Arterioscler. Thromb.,* **14:** 557-566 (1994).
38. REAVEN P. ET AL. Effects of oleate-rich and linoleate-rich diets on the susceptibility of low density lipoprotein to oxidative modification in mildly hypercholesterolemic subjects. *J. Clin. Invest.,* **91:** 668-676 (1993).
39. REAVEN, P. ET AL. Feasibility of using an oleate-rich diet to reduce the susceptibility of low-density lipoprotein to oxidative modification in

humans. *Am. J. Clin. Nutr.*, **54:** 701-706 (1991).

40. MARTIN-MORENO, J.M. ET AL. Dietary fat, olive oil intake and breast cancer risk. *Int. J. Cáncer.*, **58:** 774-780 (1994).

41. TRICHOPOULOU. A. ET AL. Consumption of olive oil and specific food groups in relation to breast cancer risk in Greece. *J. Natl. Cancer Inst.*, **87:** 110-116 (1995).

42. SZENDE, B.; TIMAR, F.; HARGITAI, B. Olive oil decroases liver damage in rats caused by carbon tetrachloride (CCl4). *Exp. Toxiool. Pathol.,* **46:** 355-359 (1994).

43. LA VECCHIA, C.; FRANCESCHI, S.; DOLARA, P. ET AL. Refined-sugar intake and the risk of colorectal cancer in humans. *Int. J. Cancer,* **55:** 386-389 (1993).

44. BOSTICK, R.M.; POTTER, J.D.; KUSHI, L.H. ET AL. Sugar, meat, and fat intake, and non-dietary risk factors for colon cancer incidence in Iowa women (United States). *Causes Control,* **5:** 38-52 (1994).

45. LENDERS, C.M.; HEDIGER, M.L.; SCHOLL, T.O. ET AL. Gestational age and infant size at birth are associated with dietary sugar intake among pregnant adolescents. *J. Nutr.,* **127:** 1113-1117 (1997).

46. LI, K.C.; ZERNICKE, R.F.; BARNARD, R.J. ET AL. Effects of a high fat-sucrose diet on cortical bone morphology and biomechanics. *Calcified Tissue International,* **47:** 308-313 (1990).

47. KATSCHINSKI, B.D.; LOGAN, R.F.; EDMOND, M. ET AL. Duodenal ulcer and refined carbohydrate intake: a case-control study assessing dietary fibre and refined sugar intake [see comments]. *Gut,* **31:** 993-996 (1990).

48. CORNEE, J.; POBEL, D.; RIBOLI, E. ET AL. A case-control study of gastric cancer and nutritional factors in Marseille, France. *Eur. J. Epidemiol.,* **11:** 55-65 (1995).

49. SAILER, D. [Does sugar play a role in the development of gastroenterologic diseases (Crohn disease, gallstones, cancer)?] *Z. Ernahrungswiss.,* **29** (Suppl. 1): 39-44 (1990).

50. MOERMAN, C.J.; SMEETS, F.W.; KROMHOUT, D. Dietary risk factors for clinically diagnosed gallstones in middle-aged men. A 25-year follow-up study (the Zutphen study). *Ann. Epidemiol.,* **4:** 248-254 (1994).

51. SAILER, D. [Does sugar play a role in the development of gastroenterologic diseases (Crohn disease, gallstones, cancer)?] *Z. Ernahrungswiss.,* **29** (Suppl. 1): 39-44 (1990).

52. SCHNOHR, P. ET AL. Egg consumption and high-density-lipoprotein cholesterol. *J. Intern. Med.,* **235:** 249-251 (1994).

53. LEVY, Y. ET AL. Consumption of eggs with meals increases the susceptibility of human plasma and low-density lipoprotein to lipid peroxidation. *Ann. Nutr. Metab.,* **40:** 243-251 (1996).

54. ZASTROW, K.D.; SCHÖNEBERG, I. [Outbreaks of food-borne infections and microbe-induced poisonings in West Germany, 1991]. *Gesundheitswesen,* **55:** 250-253 (1993).

55. LIGHTON, L.; GREENWOOD, L. Raw eggs in recipes in magazines should go. *British Medical Journal,* **308:** 595-596 (1994).

56. MISHU, B. ET AL. Salmonella enteritidis gastroenteritis transmitted by intact chicken eggs. *Ann. Intern. Med.,* **115:** 190-194 (1991).

57. DAVIGLUS, M.L. ET AL. Fish consumption and the 30-year risk of fatal myocardial infaction. *N. Eng. J. Med.,* **336:** 1046-1053 (1997).

58. CHRISTENSEN, J.H. ET AL. Effect of fish oil on heart rate variability in survivors of myocardial infarction. *British Medical Journal,* **312:** 677-678 (1996).

59. SISCOVICK, D.S. ET AL. Dietary intake and cell membrane levels of long-chain n-3 polyunsaturated fatty acids and the risk of primary cardiac arrest. *JAMA,* **274:** 1363-1367 (1995).

60. ASCHERIO, A; RIMM, E.B.; STAMPFER, M.J. ET AL. Dietary intake of marine n-3 fatty acids, fish intake, and the risk of coronary disease among men. *N. Engl. J. Med.,* **332:** 977-982 (1995).

61. PIETINEN, P.; ASCHERIO, A.; KORHONEN, P. ET AL. Intake of fatty acids and risk of coronary heart disease in a cohort of Finnish men. The Alpha-Tocopherol, Beta-Carotene Cancer Prevention Study *Am. J. Epidemiol.,* **145:** 876-887 (1997).

62. KROMHOUT, D.; BOSSCHIETER, E.B.; COULANDER, C.L. The inverse relation between fish consumption and 20-years mortality from coronary heart disease. *N. Engl. J. Med.,* **312:** 1205-1209 (1985).

63. BOEING, H.; SCHLEHOFER, B.; WAHRENDORF, J.Z. Diet, obesity and risk for renal cell carcinoma: results from a case control-study in Germany. *Ernahrungswiss,* **36:** 3-11 (1997).

64. GIOVANNUCCI, E.; RIMM, E.B.; STAMPFER, M.J. ET AL. Intake of fat, meat, and fiber in relation to risk of colon cancer in men. *Cancer Res.,* **54:** 2390-2397 (1994).

65. BINGHAM, S.A.; PIGNATELLI, B.; POLLOCK, J.R. ET AL. Does increased endogenous formation of N-nitroso compounds in the human colon explain the association between red meat and colon cancer? *Carcinogenesis,* **17:** 515-523 (1996).

66. WILLETT, W.C.; STAMPFER, M.J.; COLDITZ, G.A. ET AL. Relation of meat, fat, and fiber intake to the risk of colon cancer in a prospective study among women [see comments]. *N. Engl. J. Med.,* **323:** 1664-1672 (1990).

67. GAARD, M.; TRETLI, S.; LOKEN, E.B. Dietary fat and the risk of breast cancer: a prospective study of 25,892 Norwegian women. *Int. J. Cancer,* **63:** 13-17 (1995).

68. DE STEFANI, E.; OREGGIA, F.; RONCO, A. ET AL. Salted meat consumption as a risk factor for cancer of the oral cavity and pharynx: a case-control study from Uruguay. *Cancer Epidemiol. Biomarkers Prev.,* **3:** 381-385 (1994).

69. MACGREGOR, G.A.; SEVER, P.S. Salt-overwhelming evidence but still no action: can a consensus be reached with the food industry? *BMJ,* **312:** 1287-1289 (1996).

70. ANTONIOS, T.F.; MACGREGOR, G.A. Salt--more adverse effects. *Lancet,* **348:** 250-251 (1996).

71. JOOSSENS, J.V.; SASAKI, S.; KESTELOOT, H. Bread as a source of salt: an international comparison. *J. Am. Coll. Nutr.,* **13:** 179-183 (1994).

72. PAMPLONA ROGER, J. D. *Enciclopedia de las plantas medicinales,* Madrid, Editorial Safeliz, 5ª imp.,1998, pág. 752.

73. LUSSI, A.; JAEGGI, T.; JAEGGI-SCHARER, S. Prediction of the erosive potential of some beverages. *Caries Res.,* **29:** 349-354 (1995).

74. WEISS, G.H.; SLUSS, P.M.; LINKE, C.A. Changes in urinary magnesium, citrate, and oxalate levels due to cola consumption. *Urology,* **39:** 331-333 (1992).

75. VAN DUSSELDORP, M.; KATAN, M.B.; VAN VLIET, T. ET AL. Cholesterol-raising factor from boiled coffee does not pass a paper filter. *Arterioscler. Thromb.,* **11:** 586-593 (1991).

76. ZOCK, P.L.; KATAN, M.B.; MERKUS, M.P. ET AL. Effect of a lipid-rich fraction from boiled coffee on serum cholesterol. *Lancet,* **335:** 1235-1237 (1990).

77. WENDL, B.; PFEIFFER, A.; PEHL, C. ET AL. Effect of decaffeination of coffee or tea on gastro-oesophageal reflux. *Aliment. Pharmacol. Ther.,* **8:** 283-287 (1994).

78. HASLING, C.; SÖNDERGAARD, K.; CHARLES, P. ET AL. Calcium metabolism in postmenopausal osteoporotic women is determined by dietary calcium and coffee intake. *J. Nutr.,* **122:** 1119-1126 (1992).

79. BAK, A.A.; GROBBEE, D.E. Abstinence from coffee leads to a fall in blood pressure. *J. Hypertens. Suppl.,* **7:** S260-S261 (1989).

80. VAN DUSSELDORP, M.; SMITS, P.; THIEN, T. ET AL. Effect of decaffeinated versus regular coffee on blood pressure. A 12-week, double-blind trial. *Hypertension,* **14:** 563-569 (1989).

81. MOMAS, I.; DAURES, J.P.; FESTY, B. ET AL. Relative importance of risk factors in bladder carcinogenesis: some new results about Mediterranean habits. *Cancer Causes Control,* **5:** 326-332 (1994).

82. KUNZE, E.; CHANG-CLAUDE, J.; FRENTZEL-BEYME, R. Life style and occupational risk factors for bladder cancer in Germany. A case-control study. *Cancer,* **69:** 1776-1790 (1992).

83. WEI, M.; MACERA, C.A.; HORNUNG, C.A. ET AL. The impact of changes in coffee consumption on serum cholesterol. *J. Clin. Epidemiol.,* **48:** 1189-1196 (1995).

84. BARRACLOUGH, M.S.; BEECH, J.R. Effects of caffeine on functional asymmetry in a Posner letter-recognition task. *Pharmacol. Biochem. Behav.,* **52:** 731-735 (1995).

85. KERR, D.; SHERWIN, R.S.; PAVALKIS, F. ET AL. Effect of caffeine on the recognition of and responses to hypoglycemia in humans. *Ann. Intern. Med.,* **119:** 799-804 (1993).

86. TAVANI, A.; PREGNOLATO, A.; LA VECCHIA, C. ET AL. Coffee consumption and the risk of breast cancer. *Eur. J. Cancer Prev.,* **7:** 77-82 (1998).

87. ERNSTER, V.L.; MASON, L.; GOODSON, W.H. 3D. ET AL. Effects of caffeine-free diet on benign breast disease: a randomized trial. *Surgery,* **91:** 263-267 (1982).

88. KAWACHI, I.; COLDITZ, G.A.; STONE, C.B. Does coffee drinking increase the risk of coronary heart disease? Results from a meta-analysis. *Br. Heart J.,* **72:** 269-275 (1994).

89. DUCIMETIERE, P.; GUIZE, L.; MARCINIAK, A. Arteriographically documented coronary artery disease and alcohol consumption in French men. *The CORALI Study. Eur. Heart. J.,* **14:** 727-733 (1993).

90. CONSTANT, J. Alcohol, ischemic heart disease, and the French paradox. *Clin. Cardiol.,* **20:** 420-424 (1997).

91. YUAN, J.M.; ROSS, R.K.; GAO, Y.T. ET AL. Follow up study of moderate alcohol intake and mortality among middle aged men in Shanghai, China. *British Medical Journal,* **314:** 18-23 (1997).

92. CAMARGO, C.A; HENNEKENS, C,H.; GAZIANO, J.M. ET AL. Prospective study of moderate alcohol consumption and mortality in United States male physicians. *Arch. Intern. Med.,* **157:** 79-85 (1997).

93. RIMM, E.B.; KLATSKY, A.; GROBBEE, D. ET AL. Review of moderate alcohol consumption and reduced risk of coronary heart disease: is the effect due to beer, wine, or spirits? *British Medical Journal,* **312:** 731-736 (1996).

94. DEMROW, H.S.; SLANE, R.; FOLTS, J.D. Administration of wine and grape juice inhibits in vivo platelet activity and thrombosis in stenosed canine coronary arteries. *Circulation,* **91:** 1182-1188 (1995).

95. CONSTANT, J. Alcohol, ischemic heart disease, and the French paradox. *Clin. Cardiol.,* **20:** 420-424 (1997).

96. FRANKEL, E.N.; KANNER, J.; GERMAN, J.B. ET AL. Inhibition of oxidation of human low-density lipoprotein by phenolic substances in red wine. *Lancet,* **341:** 454-457 (1993).

97. Renaud, S.C.; Ruf, J.C. Effects of alcohol on platelet functions. *Clin. Chim. Acta,* **246:** 77-89 (1996).

98. Klatsky, A.L.; Friedman, G.D.; Siegelaub, A.B. et al. Alcohol consumption and blood presure: Kaiser-Permanente multiphasic health examination data. *N. Engl. J. Med.,* **296:** 1194-1200 (1977).

99. Criqui, M.H.; Ringel, B.L. Does diet or alcohol explain the French paradox? *Lancet.* **344:** 1719-1723 (1994).

100. Meyer, F.; White, E. Alcohol and nutrients in relation to colon cancer in middle-aged adults. *Am. J. Epidemiol.,* **138:** 225-236 (1993).

101. Ferraroni, M.; Decarli, A.; Willett, W.C. et al. Alcohol and breast cancer risk: a case-control study from northern Italy. *Int. J. Epidemiol.,* **20:** 859-864 (1991).

102. Willett, W.C.; Stampfer, M.J.; Colditz, G.A. et al. Moderate alcohol consumption and the risk of breast cancer. *N. Engl. J. Med.,* **316:** 1174-1180 (1987).

103. Falcao, J.M.; Dias, J.A.; Miranda, A.C. et al. Red wine consumption and gastric cancer in Portugal: a case-control study. *Eur. J. Cancer Prev.,* **3:** 269-276 (1994).

104. Grande, L.; Manterola, C.; Ros, E. et al. Effects of red wine on 24-hour esophageal pH and pressures in healthy volunteers. *Dig. Dis. Sci.,* **42:** 1189-1193 (1997).

105. Hernandez-Avila, M.; Colditz, G.A.; Stampfer, M.J. et al. Caffeine, moderate alcohol intake, and risk of fractures of the hip and forearm in middle-aged women. *Am. J. Clin. Nutr.,* **54:** 157-163 (1991).

106. Kaminski, M.; Franc, M.; Lebouvier, M. et al. Moderate alcohol use and pregnancy outcome. *Neurobehav. Toxicol. Teratol.,* **3:** 173-181 (1981).

107. Ducimetiere, P.; Guize, L.; Marciniak, A. Arteriographically documented coronary artery disease and alcohol consumption in French men. *The CORALI Study. Eur. Heart. J.,* **14:** 727-733 (1993).

108. Demrow, H.S.; Slane, R.; Folts, J.D. Administration of wine and grape juice inhibits in vivo platelet activity and thrombosis in stenosed canine coronary arteries. *Circulation,* **91:** 1182-1188 (1995).

109. Willett, W.C.; Ascherio, A. Trans fatty acids: are the effects only marginal? *Am. J. Public Health,* **84:** 722-724 (1994).

110. Kris-Etherton, P.M.; Shaomei, Y. Individual fatty acid effects on plasma lipids and lipoproteins: human studies. *Am. J. Clin. Nutr.,* **65** (suppl): 1628S-1644S (1997).

111. ASCN/AIN Task Force on Trans Fatty Acids. Position paper on trans fatty acids. *Am. J. Clin. Nutr.,* **63:** 663-670 (1996).

112. Kohlmeier, L.; Simonsen, N.; van't Veer, P. et al. Adipose tissue trans fatty acids and breast cancer in the European Community Multicenter Study on Antioxidants, Myocardial Infarction, and Breast Cancer. *Cancer Epidemiol. Biomarkers Prev.,* **6:** 705-710 (1997).

113. Tomomatsu, H. Health effects of oligosaccharides. *Food Tech.,* **48:** 61-65 (1994).

114. Salmeron, J.; Manson, J.E.; Stampfer, M.J. et al. Dietary fiber, glycemic load, and risk of non-insulin-dependent diabetes mellitus in women. *JAMA,* **277:** 472-477 (1997).

115. Feskens, E.J.; Virtanen, S.M.; Räsänen, L. et al. Dietary factors determining diabetes and impaired glucose tolerance. A 20-year follow-up of the Finnish and Dutch cohorts of the Seven Countries Study. *Diabetes Care,* **18:** 1104-1112 (1995).

116. Ortega, R.M.; Redondo, M.R.; Lopez-Sobaler, A.M. et al. Associations between obesity, breakfast-time food habits and intake of energy and nutrients in a group of elderly Madrid residents. *J. Am. Coll. Nutr.,* **15:** 65-72 (1996).

117. Golay, A.; Allaz, A.F.; Morel, Y. et al. Similar weight loss with low- or high-carbohydrate diets. *Am. J. Clin. Nutr.,* **63:** 174-178 (1996).

118. Valnet, J. *Traitement des maladies par les légumes, les fruits et les céréals [Treatment of diseases by vegetables, fruits and grains].* Paris, Librairie Maloine S.A. éditeur, P. 132.

119. Pamplona-Roger G. D. *Encyclopedia of Medicinal Plants.* Editorial Safeliz, Madrid, 1998, p. 160.

120. Sabate, J.; Fraser, G.E.; Burke, K. et al. Effects of Walnuts on Serum Lipid Levels and Blood Pressure in Normal Men. *The New England Journal of Medecine,* **328:** 603-607 (1993).

121. Muir, J.G.; O'Dea, K. Measurement of resistant starch: factors affecting the amount of starch escaping digestion in vitro. *American Journal of Clinical Nutrition,* **56:** 123-127 (1992).

122. Gilani, A.H.; Asif, M.; Nagra, S.A. Energy utilization of supplemented cereal diets in human volunteers. *Arch. Latinoam. Nutr.,* **36:** 373-378 (1986).

123. Watts, A.et al. Beeturia and the biological fate of beetroot pigments. *Pharmacogenetics,* **3:** 302-311 (1993).

124. Heupke, W.; Weitzel, W. *Deutsches Obst und Gemüse in der Ernährung und Heilkunde [Las frutas y hortalizas alemanas en la alimentación y en la terapéutica],* Hippokrates Verlag, Stuttgart, 1950.

125. Lampe, J.; Slavin, J.L.; Baglien, K.S. et al. Serum lipid and fecal bile acid changes with cereal, vegetable, and sugal-beet fiber feeding. *Am. J. Clin. Nutr.,* **53:** 1235-1241 (1991).

126. Song of Solomon 4: 3.

127. Mousa, O. Bioactivity of certain Egyptian Ficus species. *Journal Ethnopharmacology,* **41:** 71-76 (1994).

128. Nagy, S.; Shaw, P.E. *Tropical and subtropical fruits.* Westport (Connecticut), The AVI Publishing Company, Inc., 1980, pág. 323.

129. Osato, J.A.; Santiago, L.A.; Remo, G.M. et al. Antimicrobial and antioxidant activities of unripe papaya. *Life Sciences,* **53:** 1383-1389 (1993).

130. Satrija, F.; Nansen, P.; Bjorn, H. et al. Effect of papaya latex against Ascaris suum in naturally infected pigs. *Journal of Helminthology,* **68:** 343-346 (1994).

131. Pamplona-Roger G. D. *Encyclopedia of Medicinal Plants.* Editorial Safeliz, Madrid, 1998, p. 440.

132. Kim, M.; Shin, H.K. The water-soluble extract of chicory reduces glucose uptake from the perfused jejunum in rats. *Journal of Nutrition,* **126:** 2236-2242 (1996).

133. Helser, M.A.; Hotchkiss, J.H.; Roe, D.A. Influence of fruit and vegetable juices on the endogenous formation of N-nitrosoproline and N-nitrosothiazolidine-4-carboxylic acid in humans on controled diets. *Carcinogenesis,* **13:** 2277-2280 (1992).

134. Heyden, S. Polyunsaturated and monounsaturated fatty acids in the diet to prevent coronary heart disease via cholesterol reduction. *Ann. Nutr. Metab.,* **38:** 117-122 (1994).

135. WHO, Technical Report Series, 797. *Diet, Nutrition, and the Prevention of Chronic Diseases.* Report of a WHO Study Group. Geneva, 1990.

136. Asato, L. et al. Effect of egg white on serum cholesterol concentration in young women. *J. Nutr. Sci. Vitaminol. (Tokyo),* **42:** 87-96 (1996).

137. Oh, S.Y. et al. Eggs enriched in omega-3 fatty acids and alterations in lipid concentrations in plasma and lipoproteins and in blood pressure. *Am. J. Clin. Nutr.,* **54:** 689-695 (1991).

138. Kris-Etherton, P.M. Trans fatty acids and coronary heart disease risk. *Am. J. Clin. Nutr.,* **62:** 655S-708S (1995).

139. Fraser, G.; Sabate, J.; Beeson, L. et al. A possible protective effect of nut consumption on risk of coronary heart disease. *Archives of Internal Medecine,* **152:** 1416-1424 (1992).

Books on Health

Encyclopedia of Medicinal Plants
2 Volumes

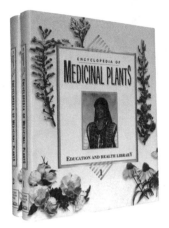

This is a complete, up-to-date, and scientific encyclopedia, based on rigorous botanical, pharmaceutical, and chemical research. More than 470 plants botanically described and classified by diseases. Numerous natural treatments are explained with clear illustrations and simple language. Numerous charts that describe the most frequent disorders and the plants that possess the active principles to correct them. 795 pages in two volumes, hardcover.

Encyclopedia of Health and Education
for the Family
4 Volumes

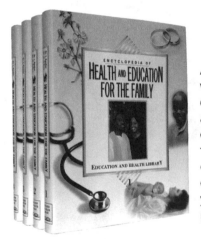

A medical-educational encyclopedia for the whole family, these books cover more than 400 diseases with their natural, pharmacological, and/or surgical treatments. The Encyclopedia contains numerous tips on educational topics for the whole family. Offering practical orientation from medics, psychologists, and educators to help you maintain and improve your physical, mental, and social health. 1,539 pages in four volumes, hardcover.

Encyclopedia of Foods and their Healing Power
3 Volumes

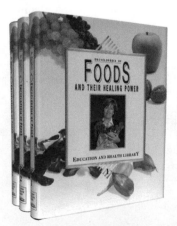

This is a modern and concise encyclopedia that presents the latest research on food science, nutrition, and dietetics. With almost 700 foods from 5 continents described and around 300 recipes, the information contained in this encyclopedia is based on the latest research at the main universities and research centers of Europe, America, and other continents. 1,278 pages in three volumes, hardcover.

For more information, write: Home Health Education Service, PO Box 1119, Hagerstown, MD, 21741-1119

MORE *FAMILY* READING

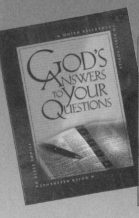

God's Answers to Your Questions
You ask the questions; it points you to Bible texts with the answers

He Taught Love
The true meaning hidden within the parables of Jesus

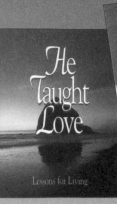

Jesus, Friend of Children
Favorite chapters from *The Bible Story*

Bible Heroes
A selection of the most exciting adventures from *The Bible Story*

The Storybook
Excerpts from Uncle Arthur's *Bedtime Stories*

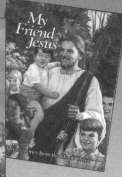

My Friend Jesus
Stories for preschoolers from the life of Christ, with activity pages

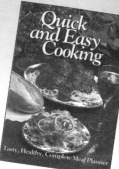

Quick and Easy Cooking
Plans for complete, healthful meals

Fabulous Food for Family and Friends
Complete menus perfect for entertaining

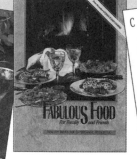

Choices: Quick and Healthy Cooking
Healthy meal plans you can make in a hurry

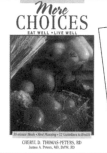

More Choices for a Healthy, Low-Fat You
All-natural meals you can make in 30 minutes

Tasty Vegan Delights
Exceptional recipes without animal fats or dairy products

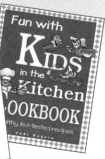

Fun With Kids in the Kitchen Cookbook
Let your kids help with these healthy recipes

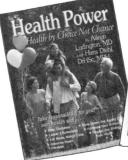

Health Power
Choices you can make that will revolutionize your health

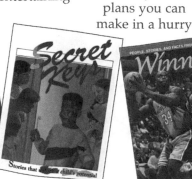

Secret Keys
Character-building stories for children

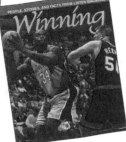

Winning
Gives teens good reasons to be drug-free

FOR MORE INFORMATION:
- mail **the attached card**
- or write
  Home Health Education Service
  P.O. Box 1119
  Hagerstown, MD 21741
- or visit **www.thebiblestory.com**